Sensual Meditation

rael

Sensual Meditation

Awakening the Mind by Awakening the Body

CONTENTS

FOREWORD BY MICHEL DEYDIER

Psychologist

If only 30 years ago someone had said that computers would revolutionize our world, nobody **would** have believed him.

In technology, as in medicine and philosophy, we have progressed far beyond the post war concepts. The human mind is developing, and so it should since it is now perceiving its environment better and better. It creates and controls its property, it discovers new energy sources and it experiments with new techniques in all fields.

The general public's reasoning has improved through its own changing culture as manifested by the conception of a more intellectual, a more sophisticated and a freer life.

But even more extraordinary is the evolution of our understanding of matter. Thanks to the efforts of our researchers, matter is becoming animate, it is getting closer to Man, it is spiritualising itself.

Previously, matter was considered to be the opposite of the mind. Today, thanks to the notable progress made in neuro-surgery and psychometric research, the activity of the brain is becoming more familiar and is losing its mystical character.

We now have information on brain functioning which puts old psychiatrical and psycho-analytical teachings right out of date.

This research never ceases to expand and, admittedly, it does worry the population; mainly because lay people make the mistake of speculating with only limited information, instead of trusting the plagiarized creative thinkers, that is to say, the researchers, beyond their hesitations and legitimate errors. For the first time in the history of our civilization, science and spirituality are walking on the same path. They both have many points in common which leave mind and matter, mental and cerebral, inseparable.

We now know, for example, which brain areas are responsible for which behaviour patterns and that the brain makes its own natural opiates (the endorphins) which are released in particular circumstances, resulting in specific emotions. Now that we know their inhibitory and excitatory properties, we can begin to understand the functioning of the brain by observing how they affect behaviour.

The biochemical activity of the human brain seems to be so automatic and autonomous that we are increasingly tempted to consider it as a social organism within itself, capable of constant self-adjustment and auto-equilibration. Thus when something goes wrong with this balanced system, the only real solution is to enhance the quality of psychosomatic integration, that is to say, to improve the connection between mind and matter.

A CLINICAL APPRAISAL OF SPIRITUAL AWAKENING:

Spiritual awakening corresponds to a state of permanent availability existing between each neuro-biological function which makes up the energetic pathways of the brain, that is to say, when all parts of the brain are communicating.

The human being who has reached an optimum level of awakening can at all times mobilize and use the various levels of processing to analyze sensory information while the ordinary person cannot function in this psychological state.

'Permanent mental analysis' precisely determines the quality of interconnection and communication between the regulation of the mind and the information received, ie, stemming from the perception of both the internal and external environment.

'Intelligence' depends on the level of regulation and integration – it is defined by the genetic code and cannot be developed beyond its ceiling level. However, it is normally not exploited as much as it could be. To operate, it requires high quality input, particularly the perception of one's internal and external world.

'Sensuality' is the capacity to perceive this environment. Sensory information is picked up through the five senses: vision, hearing, smell, touch, taste, along with the extra sense of telepathic perception.

The receptors of these senses generate pleasure and pass these images on to the central computer of the brain.

Sensuality is the most important level of processing since it provides the basic material, faithfully reproducing the information in both quality and quantity.

In order to create favourable conditions for a good mental functioning, a large number of methodologies and therapies have sprung up such as psycho-analysis, techniques of relaxation, group sessions, alpha rhythms etc.

However, until now, no technique or method has existed which is aimed at awakening the mind by awakening the body, and thus using pure sensual energy to connect and bring cerebral consciousness to a cellular level. And yet this is the keystone itself.

It is logically inconceivable to improve our permanent mental analysis without first improving our sensuality because it is this sensory information itself, coming from the external and internal environment which is the basis of every mental operation, apart from abstract thought. Every living thing possesses a sensory system, including plants, animals and humans; for without this, life itself could not be.

'Affectivity' is the complex which controls the whole of the person's emotional life. Sensory messages especially impregnate it and some are memorized.

Most of the time, affectivity acts as a support for intellectual activity. As it is deeply rooted in our unconscious, however, the faculty of reason exerts only a weak influence on unconscious elements and so it is in our interest to restore our mental and emotional order which we so desperately need, through means of our sensuality.

AWAKENING THE BODY:

Every organ and every gland of the human body is made up of cells, including the brain, the heart and the liver for example, and it is just as important for all of these organs to be, and to remain connected to the brain, so as to perceive the internal and external energetic variations. The whole of our general physiology is conditioned by 'awareness of its position in space as related to its surroundings' – a stomach which no longer knows its identity will forget part of its function and will make mistakes which will not necessarily be repaired or eliminated by the liver or the pancreas. It has been proven that most people who cannot swim would overcome their fear if they became aware of their body schema. The same applies to partial anorexics. The uses for physical awareness are unlimited and also concern everyone in perfect health who wishes to exploit his or her full potential.

The phenomenon of awakening produces a feeling of euphoria because the sensation of awareness invades us on a muscular level, reaches all of the vital organs, the respiratory and circulatory system, right even to the cellular level. It is a physiological state.

Sensual awakening gives rise to physical awakening. Sensuality along with sexuality, is part of the pleasure generating system and because of that, has been repressed for a long time, especially in our western culture.

And yet pleasure is such a natural and positive reaction. Human nature is built upon this system. In fact, the whole of biology seems to be based on this principle of pleasure. Not one action exists, both conscious or otherwise, which is done in order to avoid it. But since our morality exerts such a high level of repression, both unjustified and unjustifiable, we often follow roundabout and often unhealthy ways to achieve it. It is not by chance that a person's basic needs are directly associated with pleasure when satiated. The feeling of pleasure is not only nice, but it is also indispensable since it regulates most of our bodies' metabolic reactions, including those of our brain, and allows one to control one's own development – an awakened person knows how to enjoy his sensuality.

SENSUAL MEDITATION OR SELF-IDENTIFICATION:
Unfortunately, we cannot trigger the process of sensual and mental expansion at random or by improvising. Our sensuality has been atrophied by our affective inhibitions.

We need to relax to regulate our stress level and to satisfy our senses with colours, flavours and music... that too, is part of Man's essential needs.

Our body needs to take its bearings of the space and time which it is in, and of the space and time of which it is composed.

When we locate our body in space, we link it to our brain via awareness of our environment, which includes people. When we situate our body, organs, limbs and glands, we also link them to the brain.

When we locate our cells mentally, we link them both to our brain and to each other via the brain, since through it, each organ can become aware of its position and therefore its role within the body.

We need to feel that we are THIS, that we are HERE, and for this we must learn quite simply how to feel oneself, in other words, to identify ourselves, but not with an accepted name or socially accepted title, but purely with personal sensations. Sensual Meditation allows this and much more. Though access to it requires an initiation, or rather, a sort of reconnection with our bodily and sensual schemata, its practice remains an intimate operation. This does not mean that one must be alone to meditate. In fact, the presence of people whom we love is always positive, but it is still true that from initiation to one's 'orgasm', Sensual Meditation remains a highly personal experience in the sense that the sensations develop in a completely autarchic and self-sufficient atmosphere.

When meditating, it is as if the process of self-identification occurs automatically and it is precisely this self identification which carries us towards knowing ourselves.

The state of awakening is a state of mind in which creativity flourishes and what is more, it vastly improves the quality or our inter-human relationships. Meditating is not a complicated operation, one must first learn to encourage those sensations which eventually lead to the expansion of consciousness. As euphoria begins to penetrate into the body tissues, so does the proliferation of the muscular and nerve connections.

Then during everyday life between meditations, a psychological and physical well-being instills itself which adds a new dimension to life.

Sensual Meditations' depth of understanding as taught by Rael, answers all of modern psychology's deficiencies because it allows the awakening of the mind, the awakening of the body, and the fulfilment of sensuality.

It regulates our affectivity by reducing any frustrations while preserving our emotional life.

It gives rise to a phenomenon of natural re-equilibration of our metabolic system without any external intervention of medical drugs.

It is accessible to everyone.

It possesses, in my opinion, highly valuable curative and preventative qualities.

PREFACE BY DR. PAUL AUGER

Psychiatrist

Sensual Meditation as taught by Rael is useful for all types of people, particularly for the people of today.

Basically, it aims at awakening the mind by awakening the body. It is more than just a technique of relaxation, even though it uses, as do most others, an heightened oxygenation of the blood. The background music is appropriately suggestive and gently induces tranquillity and peace.

Sensual Meditation also has the added advantage of 'rendering conscious': of bringing the vital and functional presence of the various tissues and specific cells composing them, to the cerebral cortex, in a relatively short time.

It seeks the admiring and marvelling awareness of the infinitely small, down to the biochemical level, and its position relative to and harmonious with the body as a whole. By inviting, or rather by inciting, the nerves and their 'neuro-transmitters' to transmit adequately their organic messages to the cerebral cortex, it is able to increase self esteem, and catalyse sensual enjoyment. This is directly complimentary with science and the two together can create, interactively, a planetary awareness. In my opinion, it is in this way that Sensual Meditation can awaken Mankind's search for enjoyment and can prevent adrenalin and other such toxic derivatives from reaching the brain. The human brain is a complex gland, both perfected and perfectioning, fulfilling the enjoyment of the senses through perception of the infinitely large. The spiral opens the way to the fourth dimension of time and perhaps its contraction is speed.

In a nutshell, Sensual Meditation, through a biochemical process lasting only a few minutes at a time, allows Man to see other humans as his brothers, and to taste and feel part of the universal harmony which is both created and creator.

INTRODUCTION

Rael is the young journalist who you have seen numerous times on television, relating both his contacts with extra- terrestrials, and his journey to their planet in one of their machines, what Man calls 'flying saucers'.

These people from the other planet, or rather, the Elohim, as they are called, entrusted Rael with a series of extra- ordinary messages which have been published in French as three books entitled *Le Livre Qui Dit La Vérité*, *Les Extra- Terrestres M'ont Emmené Sur Leur Planete* and *Accueillir Les Extraterrestres, Ils Ont Créé L'humanité en Laboratoire*. These have been published as two books entitled; 'The Message Given By Extra-Terrestrials' and 'Let's Welcome the Extra- Terrestrials'.

Among other things, the messages explain how these people had landed on Earth, and through progressive experiments in genetic engineering, had created all life on Earth including 'Man in their image'. They also relate how all the religious texts of the major religions of this world, including The Bible, in fact describe this scientific creation. In the Old Testament, one repeatedly finds the word 'Elohim', for example in Genesis – 'in the beginning, the spirit of Elohim flew over the waters', or 'The first day, Elohim did this', 'The second day, Elohim did that', etc. By comparing the different versions of The Bible you can see for yourself that what was originally the ancient Hebrew word 'Elohim', meaning literally: 'Those who came from the sky,' has now been translated into the word 'God'. That is to say, what was originally a plural, has now been changed to a singular. However, some more honest translators who knew full well that 'Elohim' meant 'Those who came from the sky', kept the word as a plural instead of falsely translating it as 'God', which is why one can still find this plural word 'Elohim' in some versions of The Bible, such as those translated by Edouard Dhorme.

Under this new light, it is easier to understand where it is written: 'And Elohim created Man in their image', especially now that our scientists are beginning to synthesize DNA and will soon create other 'men in our image'. It becomes even more obvious when we consider how the exploits of flying something which is heavier than air dates back only to the beginning of this century, and for our primitive ancestors, anything coming from the sky just had to be divine. There are still to this day people on a Pacific island adoring empty Coca Cola cans and chewing-gum packets, waiting for the return of the 'white sky gods and their metal birds'. The Americans had in fact used the island as an air-base when fighting against Japan, but since the end of the war when they packed up and went, the 'Cargo Cult' started, with the natives desperately awaiting anything made in the USA to drop from the sky.

But the books containing the messages from those people who had created the first humans in a laboratory not only constitute a fantastic demystification of all religions, but also bring an equally fabulous set of techniques for human fulfilment, called Sensual Meditation. The thousands of people associating with Rael, and helping him to spread and publicize these prodigious messages, were able to experience for themselves the marvellous results of these meditation techniques, following the courses of awakening organized during August at various camp-sites around the world, and they now wish to make this available to everyone, by setting up permanent centres of pleasure, awakening and fulfilment. Furthermore, there were many who wished to benefit from this teaching, or at least its basis, in their own time and in their own home, in order to re-harmonize themselves after a stressful day, or even to progress further in their own development and fulfilment. It was in this context that the present work and the basic programme of meditation CDs and audio cassettes was born.

1

THE WATCHMAKER'S INSTRUCTION MANUAL

Happy is the one who has pierced the mystery of things VIRGIL

The symbol (see left, below) which adorned the cover of the original edition of this book might have shocked you. Rest assured, it had nothing to do with the criminal against humanity who stole the central part, the swastika, and made it the emblem of one of the worst genocides in the history of our planet.

In fact the whole symbol represents infinity in time and space. The triangle pointing down represents the infinitely small and the triangle pointing upwards, the infinitely large – obviously, they are both linked. As for the swastika in the centre, it represents infinity in time which, quite obviously, is applicable to both the infinitely small and large.

Thanks to their 25,000 year scientific advance on us, the Elohim have been able to prove that the particles of the atoms which make us up are universes in which one can find planets, on which live intelligent people just like us, and who themselves are composed of atoms whose particles are universes, etc.

From there, they were able to prove that the stars of our universe are what make up a particle of a huge atom located somewhere in an intelligent living being, who is perhaps contemplating its own planet's sky, wondering if there is any intelligent life elsewhere in its universe, a universe which is also but a particle of an atom.

The Elohim, these people from space who created us in their laboratory, also discovered that time is inversely proportional to the mass of the universe which it is passing – that is to say, to continue the previous example, during what is for us one second, thousands of years have passed by for the people living on a planet in our big toe, whereas the amount of time equivalent to one of our life-spans is but a fraction of a second for the gigantic being of which our planet is but a particle of one of its atoms.

Obviously, for people who have reached such a level of civilization where they are capable of creating living beings in a laboratory with, as the Scriptures say, 'a handful of dust', that is to say, the chemicals contained in the soil of our planet, the characteristics of their creations which they decide to design can vary infinitely. Whether it be the colours of butterfly wings or the shape of a flower's petals, all this is easy for the Elohim to programme into the genetic code of the species which they are designing.

What is applicable to the physical characteristics of the individual is also applicable to their mental characteristics.

Most recently, we have been able to modify animal behaviour in the laboratory by acting on the chemical reactions within the parts of the brain which determine behaviour, and thus make wolves fearful and lambs fierce. And human science is only just beginning in this area.

If we were to create an animal in a laboratory, first of all we would give it its physical aspects, then we must decide upon its mental characteristics. The latter will obviously influence its appearance since if we decided to create a herbivore we would have to think about giving it a dentition fit for grazing.

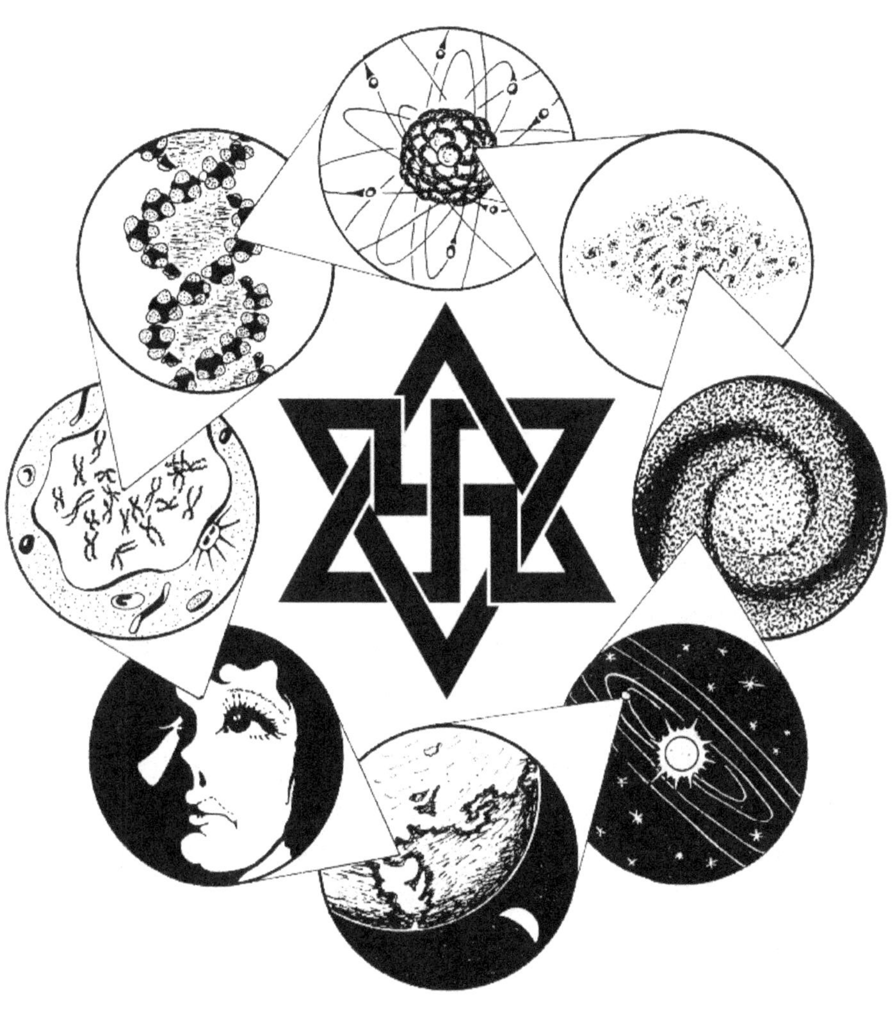

In the centre of the image, you can see the symbol of infinity, one of the oldest symbols on our planet. It appears in the "Tibetan Book of the Dead", or "Bardo Thodol" and was known in several ancient cultures. It is also the symbol of the Elohim civilisation and is the original symbol of the Raelian Movement. The star of David represents infinity in space, while the swastika inside symbolises infinity in time.

If we wished it to live in a region with a very cold climate we must also think about giving it thick fur, and if it is to live in the snow and other carnivores exist in the same region which would make it too much of an easy prey, then we must make it such that its fur becomes an immaculate white during these dangerous periods.

As far as reproduction is concerned, we must think about giving the animal the organs necessary for the growth of the 'organized cancer', or rather, the living cells which one day will develop in the mother's womb into another similar animal – a faithful reproduction.

We must also determine that at a certain time of the year our female animal secretes certain substances which give off a particular smell to attract the male so that copulation can occur, and obviously the male himself will have been given olfactory sensors linked to certain centres in his brain which trigger in him the desire for copulation.

It is already well established that certain female moths emit a smell which the male can smell several kilometres away, which shows the quality of its 'nose'.

Thus we have just seen how we would trigger the desire to copulate in the male and female animal that we wish to make. Next, we must ensure that the act of copulation itself triggers off pleasurable reactions in the brain of both partners so that with the help of the Pavlovian reflex, they would wish to do it again. For this, their sexual organs must be equipped with nerve endings to transmit the stimulation to the brain and trigger the feelings of pleasure.

Thus the contact area on the male and female sexual organs must be large enough for the pleasurable sensation to be strong.

And so we see that the mental characteristics linked to the functioning of our animal determine to a large extent its physical characteristics.

It is important to understand clearly that these characteristics, mental, physical and those related to the behaviour of the animal that we are planning on constructing are all programmed by composing the sequence of the genetic code. This is exactly comparable to the fact that the way the letters of the alphabet are ordered when I write, give either long, hard-to-read phrases or short and clear ones, technical and hermetic, or poetic and enthusiastic – and with the same letters of the alphabet it is possible to trigger reactions of disgust, sexual desire or salivation, etc. in the reader.

Instead of ordering letters in a certain way, we can use atoms and molecules which, depending on the sequence in which they are ordered, will result in the animal having two wings or four legs, or be a herbivore or a carnivore, viviparous or oviparous etc...

This genetic phrase which every living creature possesses, is called the genetic code in science, whereas certain esoteric traditions refer to it as the 'name of each animal', a name which is its own and to which it 'answers'.

Thus we have seen that when building a living being we can design the physical characteristics that we wish as well as its mental characteristics, in other words, its desires, mannerisms and habits.

When the Elohim designed life on Earth, they created an immense variety of animals and plants by balancing the desires and reproductive systems of these creatures so that the whole was capable of reproducing and surviving for as long as the environment remained the same as when they first designed it.

To use contemporary fashionable words, one could say that the group of plants and animals as a whole which was created in a laboratory on Earth by the Elohim had to be ecologically balanced. The plants allow the herbivores to nourish themselves, which are themselves eaten by the carnivores, which, when they multiply too much, do not find enough food and so, being weak, die, generally of an epidemic. With few predators surviving these epidemics, the herbivores are then free to multiply again in large numbers, which gives the remaining predators plenty to eat, and the cycle continues indefinitely. This succession of disequilibria which alternately compensate themselves, represents an ecological balance as a whole which makes the totality of the creation viable.

When the Elohim finally decided to create people similar to themselves 'in their image', as it says in The Bible, they created humans with the identical physical appearance and mental characteristics as themselves. Who knows more about the watch than the watchmakers themselves? No one, obviously.

Thus it is clear that all of the human's mental characteristics were given to him on purpose by those who created him, and therefore the best method of utilizing these capabilities can come only from the designers themselves, as an 'instructions for use' manual.

While on the subject, it is important to underline the difference between Man and animals. Animals automatically develop and fulfil themselves in their environment for the simple reason that they were designed to develop and blossom in their natural habitat but not to modify it. Man, on the other hand, was designed to change the environment. In fact, animals were designed ready made with their tastes and desire which they are incapable of questioning whereas Man is capable of changing all his habits on every level.

For example, as far as their habitat is concerned, robin red breasts have always built their nests in the same way, and will always continue to do so, whereas man went from mud huts to sky scrapers, going through intermediary stages such as thatched roofs and igloos.

It is precisely this superior intelligence which characterizes humans which is the root cause of the difficulty they have in fulfilling themselves and blossoming naturally.

When a bird has slept well, eaten well and is cleaning its feathers in the sun, it is automatically in total harmony. It has reached its true potential and has nothing else to do. It is natural for it to feel 'high' and it automatically feels good all over because it is programmed never to question itself as far as its behaviour and way of life are concerned. Birds, like all animals, are specifically programmed computers.

Man on the other hand, never ceases to question himself and has never ceased to do so ever since he first existed, and that is why he is a creator. Once he has slept well and eaten well, he will start thinking about ways of accumulating food to see him through difficult times, and once that is done, he will give himself to another task, and then another, never ceasing to question and re-evaluate himself at all levels. Even if we were to imagine people who had everything that they needed to live with for their whole life in terms of both housing and food, they would still launch themselves into more and more astounding enterprises, whether these be artistic creations done for the love of art, or the creation of enterprises designed to increase their fortune, or simply so as to have an 'occupation'.

Be it in his habitat, food, work, leisure or even sexuality, Man always seeks change, and this is purely because Man, in contrast to animals, was designed as a self-programmable computer; that is to say capable at all times of questioning, re-evaluating and reconsidering his habits, traditions and morals. Even though Man's ability to re-evaluate himself continually represents an enormous superiority over animals, and though he must develop this capacity to the full in order to reach full awakening, it is also necessary for him to situate himself regularly according to his environment, that is to say, to realize where 'he is at' relative to his circumstances.

Being aware of what we are precisely at the time of doing this exercise provides us with moments of ecstasy and allows us to be subsequently even more efficient in our capacity to use our auto-reprogramming abilities. This momentary break in Humanity's frantic race of continual reassessment and self- questioning can be compared to when a bird settles on its branch, enjoying a ray of sunshine and sings for no other reason than for the joy of singing.

This is part of the 'instructions for use' for the fantastic machines that we are, which the maker is giving to us now that our level of civilization allows us to understand and use them.

Who better than the watchmaker can tell us how to make the watch work? Sensual Meditation, revealed by these people who had come previously from their distant planet to create us in a laboratory, is the simplest and most efficient set of techniques for human awakening and fulfilment, for the plain and simple reason that it is given to us by those who designed us as we are.

Certainly, many other techniques now exist, most of them coming from the East, which a long time ago the Elohim had revealed to certain prophets or initiates such as Buddha or other Tibetan monks, but those teachings had been given to primitives who were still dominated by completely absurd superstitions and beliefs, and who, most of them, badly or only partially understood the Elohim's teachings and had almost entirely distorted them while passing them on to their disciples. Most often, the teachings revealed by the Elohim were mixed together with the primitive beliefs of the times, producing religions which conserved some excellent methods of awakening, but were unfortunately drowned by an oppressive mysticism and an atrophying ritualism.

The original teachings, rediscovered thanks to the recent messages of the Elohim, represent a return to the source, allowing us to understand the concrete basis of all these oriental techniques, which themselves serve as further evidence of the way our creators, from the beginning, have been consistently helping us to improve the living conditions of the creation that they love as their own children – Humanity.

Furthermore, it is important to add that a person cannot be totally in harmony if he still mentally harbours false and generally guilt-inducing concepts, arising from primitive and therefore mystical concepts of the universe. This is why certain exercises, themselves excellent, but taught by organizations from the East, found their beneficial effects partially or totally inhibited by the mystical context which in the end almost completely invaded the original teaching.

Sensual Meditation allows us to rediscover the techniques of awakening, free from the handicap of centuries-old theological encrustation.

A return to the watchmaker's 'instruction manual'.

2

THE STAGES TOWARDS
TOTAL AWAKENING

The path which leads to total awakening comprises several stages which can be passed only in a certain order. We cannot climb the top step of a staircase without having first put our feet on the first step.

The first step of this staircase is called 'the sudden dawning', where it dawns upon us, or where we realize, how mediocre our life is, how mediocre and how lacking in precision our objectives are. We get the feeling of having wasted our time during the course of our life, of having run after diplomas, money, the ideal partner, etc... and suddenly we find ourselves playing out a role in Society or even in the family, a role which we would never have wished to take, if we had 'had the choice'.

Once this realization of dissatisfaction has hit us, and it follows that in your case it has since otherwise you would not be reading these lines, the next step is that of 'information.' When we realize that something seems to be wrong with our life, it is usually due to a 'trigger event' stemming from a thirst for information. This trigger event can be the meeting of someone who lives differently from our norm, or what we thought was the best way to live, and yet who seems to be happier than us. Alternatively, it could be the discovery of a book or a film in which what we thought was absolutely unquestionably true suddenly seems not quite so true.

This 'trigger event', this beneficial accident, produces in us the realization of how possible it is for us to live differently, to think in a different way from how we usually do – and even if it may at first sight seem shocking that certain principles drummed into us by our upbringing are being questioned, we still wish to find out more, even if it is just to see if those who live outside 'our' norm can really be happy and if their smile might not be hiding despair and anxiety.

That is when it is important really to inform ourselves without any preconceived ideas and above all, without trusting the slanderous gossip coming from people who aren't strong enough to question themselves and who thus prefer to make fun of that which they are afraid of understanding for fear of consequently being even more unhappy than they usually are. Weakness, fear and unhappiness, that is what the minds of those who live tied to their traditions are full of, that is to say, full of habits and superstitions coming from the primitives who preceded us and for whom everything which was unexplained just had to be miraculous, divine or... diabolical... A comet, a black cat, a solar eclipse, everything was a pretext or mysterious signal hailing and forecasting bad luck, since for them everything was a portent of good or bad. Now that we know how to analyze scientifically and explain clearly everything around us, now that we know how to create life in the laboratory, travel into outer space, modify animal behaviour or colour, enable the blind to see thanks to electronic prostheses, now that we can understand all these things, we can realize how ridiculous all these superstitions are, and yet we are still brought up, educated and conditioned by them.

That is why, even now that Man walks on the moon, the election of a new Pope makes all the headlines, films about black-magic are the best sellers and the Americans have processions to make the rain fall during times of drought...

But since you have chosen really to inform yourself and without a biased point of view, you have begun really to understand by yourself how ridiculous this superstitious and uninformed situation is, which the governments carefully cultivate, since it is in their interest for the populace not to ask too many questions...

But let us return to our work programme.

Once we have informed ourselves, and it is this stage which we will go through in the next chapter, then a new realization will dawn upon us as we elevate our level of global awareness; a realization which will allow us to see to what extent what we used to take for granted as completely natural was, in fact, only the result of the way we were conditioned by our education. Then will come the third step, probably the most important, and to which we will certainly have to return during various circumstances of our life when faced with events which we had not taken into account during our organized clearing out of the refuse of received ideas.

This third step is the organization of a great spring-cleaning of all that controls our behaviour. It is a 'brain-washing' which we carry out on ourselves to clean out from this organ all the elements which have been stuffed in pell-mell and which have caused both our more obvious inhibitions as well as those which we are not even aware of ourselves and so which are more annoying and dangerous.

Briefly, it consists of questioning deeply all of our actions and reactions so as to become aware of and define those which are due to our educators and those which stem from our very own selves, and then eliminating the former if they are in contradiction with our deepest tastes and aspirations.

After having emptied ourselves of all our conscious and unconscious conditioning, which, though we might not realize it, influence all our tastes, likes and dislikes, we can then reach the fourth step where we will try to reprogram ourselves according to our own wishes, and this time not having to listen to, and owing nothing to our educators, parents, or even the interference of our environment. We will reprogram ourselves simply by discovering our real and strictly personal and individual tastes, likes and dislikes.

Once we have eliminated the elements which caused the taboos within us, this wilful and voluntary reprogramming can be done by becoming aware of our sensuality, that is to say by the optimal usage of our senses, through which our whole being is linked to the infinite surrounding us and of which we are made up.

Then we will be ready to tackle the last stage which is the one from which the infinite staircase rises, leading to total awakening through a global awareness of space and time, resulting in a higher level of consciousness and allowing those who reach it to live in a permanent state of total harmony.

But... let us start at the beginning and be careful not to stumble on the first step!

3

BECOMING AWARE OF ONESELF

The education that we have received has conditioned us without us being aware of it, and has made of us people pulled between two tendencies hypocritically confused by our educators – the belief in 'God' with Man being the fruit of a supernatural creation on the one hand, and on the other, the scientific dogma stating that we are the fruit of a slow evolution due to an unimaginable succession of chance mutations and that our grandfather was a monkey... In fact, there are many 'scientists' who back evolution during the week and then go to church on Sunday morning. And if, as a child, you had the misfortune and sacrilegious audacity to have had the 'wicked' idea of asking 'Why?', nine times out of ten you would have been told to finish your soup and shut up... Why? Simply because your educators themselves were torn between a sacrosanct tradition which they had to pass on to their descendants at all costs and a so-called scientific reasoning which through no virtue of its own, is now considered to be irrefutable by the higher 'authorities' who decide to impose such dogmas.*

* It is important to note that some scientists are beginning to doubt the theory of evolution, and that an American university is teaching the possibility that life could have been created. A book entitled 'Evolution or Creation' shows to what extent the dogma of evolution can be shown as illogical and unscientific. See the bibliography at the end of this book.

THE TOTAL AWAKENING SCALE

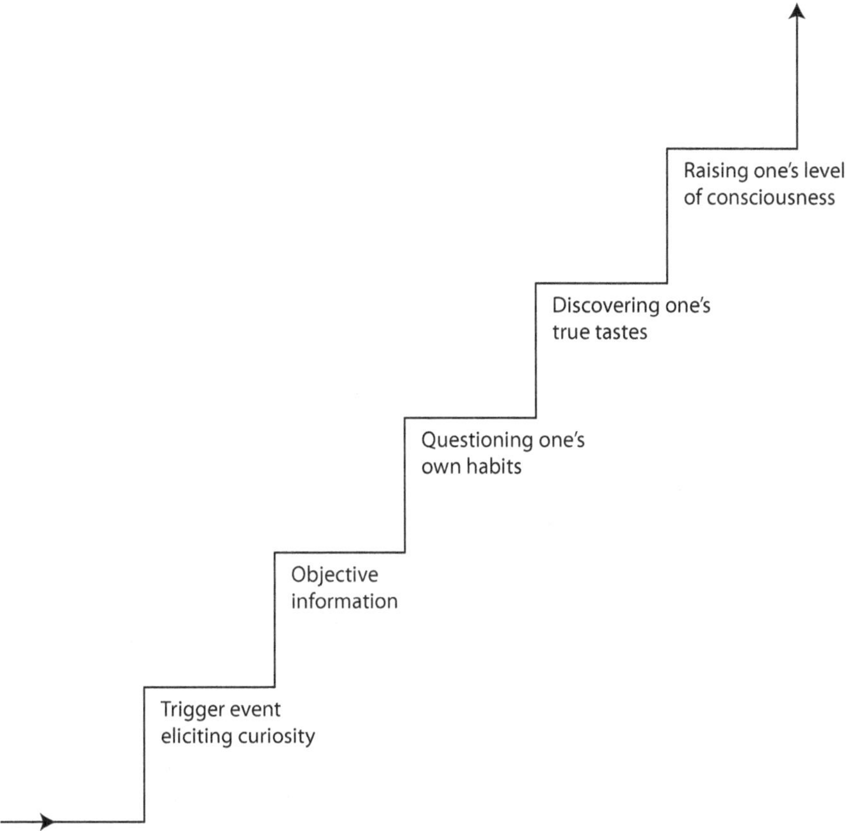

How do you expect that living among all of this, your own educators are not themselves unbalanced and ill at ease with themselves? And if an educator is not at ease with himself, it is inevitable that he passes on his fears to those whom he is forming (in this case it would be more exact to say 'deforming').

The fact of discovering that we are the fruit of an intelligent decision, that we were designed scientifically by people coming from another planet, and that they created us in their own image, ie, capable of understanding where we came from, why we are here, and what we can become – the act of discovering all this changes the whole basis of the problem.

And what is more, as was mentioned earlier, we are lucky enough to have been given the 'instruction manual' on how to make us tick, by the watch makers themselves!

But before talking about the instructions, let us look at what the clock really is and how it works.

The Huming Being – A Biological Computer, Self-Reprogrammable And Self-Reproducing

We are nothing other than a computer, a sort of machine whose performance capacities are only relatively mediocre when compared to some objects made by humans.

For a machine to function, it must first be capable of feeding itself with energy. When we are hungry, we stop working and we feed ourselves to build up our strength. British researchers have designed a metal robot which works all day as a sort of pickup-truck. When its batteries are flat, the machine stops working, and equipped with it own wheels and a camera, directs itself to a source of electricity and plugs in to recharge itself. It 'feeds' itself just like us, and when its batteries are sufficiently recharged, it unplugs itself and starts to work again. Thus we can see that the capacity of feeding oneself with energy when the need is felt, does not constitute a superiority of man over machine. Furthermore, work is now being done on robots fed by solar energy, capable of storing it up for use during the rainy season which will allow it to work without having to stop to feed itself. In fact, Man is not capable of feeding himself with solar energy which is already a first inferiority of Man compared to machines in the field of power source.

Let's now see whether sight makes us superior. We have just mentioned that some robots are equipped with cameras for them to 'see' with, so that they can move about without bumping into obstacles just as we do. These cameras are linked to the robot's computer which analyze the transmitted images in exactly the same way that our brain does.

Still no superiority of man over machines in sight. What is more, we could easily equip our robot computer with multiple lenses cameras, one of them being a zoom lens allowing it to see several miles away, another being a wide angled lens allowing it to see wide areas in one go, another being a microscope allowing it see into the infinitely small and another fitted to see infrared so that it can see at night... Such a simultaneous and instantaneous performance is impossible for the human being who has to use binoculars, a concave lens, a microscope, or infrared glasses to get the same effect and which in any case, cannot all be looked through at the same time... Yet another superiority of machine over man.

Let's take another sense, that of hearing. You all know that we perceive only a small percentage of the sounds around us, but dogs can pick up ultra and infra sounds, and we can equip a robot with ultra and infra sound receptors. What is more, it can also be designed to detect the precise direction from which the sound is coming, as well as its distance from the sound source. We are incapable of such precise skills. The same goes for the sense of smell.

It is impossible for us to analyze the chemical constituents of a smell – all we can do is to say 'it smells good' or 'it smells bad.' The robot, on the other hand, can be designed to analyze instantaneously the chemical constituents of the surrounding smells, to calculate the distance and direction of their source, and even to say whether they are dangerous to man, even if Man cannot smell them himself.

As far as the sense of touch goes, we are just as limited. When we touch something, all we can say is 'it's hot' or 'it's cold', or even 'it's hard' or 'it's soft', which, let's face it, is pretty vague. The robot's computer however, can measure the precise weight, hardness and temperature of what it touches using its prehensile senses, the equivalent of human hands.

Finally, our sense of taste is also limited to the extent that we can say only 'it's sweet', 'it's salty', 'it tastes good' or 'it tastes bad', allowing us to swallow gullibility any old fish so long as it has been seasoned sufficiently to excite our palate. On the other hand, the computer can be equipped with chemical analyzers so as to name the exact constituents of the sub- stance, even though the only use it can have for this ability is not for itself, since it can feed directly from the sun's rays, but to help humans by informing them about what they are eating.

Thus we can see how a simple machine is not only not inferior to Man, but is capable of being given infinitely superior characteristics.

All that is left is the sixth sense, extra-sensory perception, an ability which humans almost never use and which a computer could also use much better. Information trans- mission without the use of the five ordinary senses happens every day thanks to radio communication and equipping our robot with a radio emitter-receiver for it to communicate with other robots would be child's play. So, to conclude, we can say that everything that Man does, a computer can do better. But when it becomes obvious that our sensory characteristics are very limited, maybe you will say that Man's 'divine essence' must reside elsewhere. In his memory? Impossible! As you know, any old pocket computer can store in its memory far more information than can any of our academics, and moreover, can recall it instantaneously without making any mistakes. Computerization, which is increasingly becoming part of our environment, proves it to us every day: pocket calculators, pocket translators containing the equivalent of an eight language dictionary, electronic opponents to play chess with us at international championship level...

And yet this is only the beginning of computerization. Each year, electronic components double their capabilities.

Some people are already considering the possibility of storing all of Humanity's knowledge in all disciplines in just one crystal just a few millimetres small!

This book that you are reading was written directly onto a disk linked to a revolutionary computerized system, but which will in only a few months, be out of date. And yet, on a small disk, the size of a 45RPM record, one can store all the information, every word and every letter of two books like this one.

Thus so far no sign of a 'divine essence' in all this, nor of any human characteristics which cannot be replaced.

What about the ability to create works of art? Not even in that! Already now, computerized composers exist which compose music and play it. Everyone has heard what synthesizers sound like, which are used more and more in popular music. All it is, is a computer capable of reproducing the sound characteristics of every instrument, even the human voice. This machine can be programmed to play a piece of Mozart or Bach with much more precision than any symphony orchestra in the world. Imagine an orchestra with 100 violins. Never will those 100 violins play the music all exactly in time together. There will always be a time gap of a few tenths of a second between the promptest and the last musicians and a few hundredths of a second between each musician. The computer however, can synthesize the sound of 100 violins and can make them all play together exactly to the millisecond, much better than any conductor could ever achieve with human musicians.

Some people might say that it is precisely that little time delay between musicians which gives the spice and personality of each conductor but this hesitation itself can be programmed to give the computer a personality identical to the conductor.

Yet another advantage of the computer synthesizer is that it can produce much purer sounds than the archaic instruments which have to rely upon the natural acoustics of the room in which they are used. This is particularly noticeable when during recordings, the sound is distorted by the room's acoustics and then has to pass through a microphone and amplifier to be recorded, and then passed through an amplifier and loudspeaker to be heard. The synthesizer on the other hand, can send almost totally pure sounds directly to the amplifier without these being in the least bit distorted by the acoustic faults of the room in which it is being played. As composer Jean Claude Risset, in charge of CNRS research, said: 'there is no limit to the computer which can play difficult pieces and complex rhythms with a precision unattainable by human musicians – and some musicians even wish to use computers simply so as to dispense with musicians.'

What is possible with sounds is also possible with shapes, colours, perfumes and tastes.

The painter who draws the curves of a hip is simply drawing an ideal line relative to the numerous other possible lines. The computer can do this too including the defects which characterize certain painters like Modigliani who adorns his subjects with long necks, or Buffet who draws with a maximum number of vertical lines. This the computer can do with ease. In the same way that it can play a piece of music in Bach's style, so can it paint a subject in the same way as Modigliani.

A computer can even find a style which does not exist, by scanning all those which do and designing one corresponding to the public's taste. 'The role of the computer in the process of creativity is still in its infancy and is already very promising.' It was Arnold Kaufman from the National Polytechnic Institute of Grenoble who said that and the immediate future will surpass his predictions.

Computers are already capable of creating images, composing music, synthesizing smells and drawing architecture etc...

We have to face it, even in creativity, man is not superior to machines.

What is left? The capacity to reproduce? Not even that. It is easy to envisage the designing of computers programmed to build other computers in their image, capable of creating more of themselves etc, thus designing a 'species' capable of proliferating and multiplying.

Thus nothing about Man is impossible to reproduce mechanically, and therefore Man is not superior to machines. In fact, we have just seen that Man's performance is fairly mediocre compared to what is technically possible.

Man is simply a biological computer, self-programming and self-reproducing, lost in the infinitely large, composed of the infinitely small and making up and made up from eternity. The only superiority of man over machines is his capacity to decide whether or not he will build those computers which will be at his service, and decide what their limits shall be. In fact he could even give them abilities far superior to his own and even programme them to become the dominant species on Earth, which will eventually destroy its own creators. It all depends on how they will be programmed. However, it seems reasonable to programme them so as to obey us and serve us efficiently.

But have we therefore no superiority over machines? And what about the 'soul' you might ask? As we have seen at the start of this book, since the universe is infinite, there can be no centre which proves the existence of a 'God,' and since those who did create us did it in a laboratory using a perfect grasp of genetics, the soul does not exist either. Soon, when our most advanced scientists create a 100 per cent synthetic human being, it will prove definitively that there is no soul. However though there is no god, there is infinity which is in us just as we are in it, which is eternal. And if in your mind, that was your definition of the word 'God', then you were not wrong. But be careful. Infinity couldn't care less whatever your actions may be, whether you are altruistic, or murder

1,000 people, it does not mind, for the good and simple reason that infinity has no consciousness of its own, being both everywhere and nowhere.

To return to the soul, if to you it means 'that which gives someone their own individuality or personality', (following back the etymology of the French word 'ame' to its Latin 'anima', meaning 'that which animate') then we are talking about the genetic code. And in the light of some of the most recent scientific experiments, we notice that it is possible to recreate a living being starting from one of its cells, a process which genetic engineering calls 'cloning', just as the Elohim, those people from space who created us in their image, told us. Therefore it will soon be possible to recreate someone after they have died by using the genetic code from one of their preserved cells.

But if to you the soul is an ethereal vapour which floats gently away after death and which constitutes our real personality, then you will have to resign yourself to abandoning this primitive and destabilizing concept since, as do all these false ideas, it creates a duality between the mind and the body, by considering the body to be in one place while the mind is supposed to be elsewhere, doing something else... Surely those who created us are best placed to know whether or not they designed us with something resembling an ethereal soul. They say that there isn't one and prove it by being able to create 50 copies of the same person through cloning in the laboratory. If no one intervenes after death to recreate the dead person using his genetic code, then the matter which made up this person will disperse and the person will no longer exist. 'From dust you came and to dust you will return.'

Therefore, since the soul does not exist, it cannot be considered a superiority of man over machine. But the genetic code, does represent a superiority over a robot's metal computer. Every cell of a living being, whether it be the cell of the hand or foot, contains the information to recreate the whole being. But if we take a bit of a robot's 'claw', we cannot find any information allowing us to rebuild the whole robot again, not unless the robot is biological... What is a biological robot? It is a robot which instead of being made of metal, is made of living matter just like us.

To summarize, we have just seen how we are simply machines of modest performance, but able to surround our selves with machines which are both superior to us and which we designed so as to give us time to create and fulfil ourselves. This will be our privilege only if we decide to make it so; it will not happen by itself.

Once we are able to remove all the mystery surrounding us and remove those attitudes which consider that our human characteristics are sacred, unintelligible and transcendent, then we can begin to see clearer and get a better idea of ourselves. Thus we become aware that we are part of the Infinite with very limited capabilities.

But even though these capabilities might be extremely limited, they still allow us to feel the infinity around us so that we can situate ourselves relative to it, and if we know how, these capabilities enable us to put ourselves in harmony with it.

Before closing this chapter, which is designed to destroy in us all false ideas about ourselves, one thing still remains. This is to demystify the act which primitives are so desperate to render sacrosanct, either through ignorance, or more likely by playing on the ignorance of the masses to whom these religions are aimed, and that is 'the creation of life'. This is the 'mystery' which is the last remaining bastion which ministers of the 'cults of the uncultured' shelter behind.

In fact the creation of life is not a mystery at all, and it is not by chance that the religions who continue to proclaim that it is a mystery, are losing more and more of their 'faithful' and consequently have to lead vast publicity campaigns in countries where there is over 90 per cent illiteracy. In this way, they try to compensate for their losses of members in the educated West by trying to get converts in the uneducated countries which are hardly informed about scientific discoveries at all. Therefore the Pope has to travel to South America, the Middle East etc...

What is in fact the creation of life in a mother's womb? Well, simply the creation of a new genetic code, a new 'genetic phrase' as we described it earlier. We have seen that every living thing has a 'name' whose letters are atoms and molecules. When a living organism is made in a laboratory, a new 'name' is created by assembling the atoms and molecules in a certain way, and if this organism is to be human, its 'genetic name' will be composed of 45 'syllables', which we call 'chromosomes.' If this organism, as is the case here, is capable of sexual reproduction, then it will give half of its 'genetic name' which is its own personal phrase, to the egg and when its partner of the opposite sex gives the other half of the genetic code, it will be fertilized and become their child. Thus they will each give 23 chromosomes, one half through the sperm, the other through the egg which when assembled, will form a cell containing a total of 46 chromosomes. The first cell of this new living being will then divide into two cells, then four, eight, etc... until one day it will be born, and eventually become a man or a woman.

Nothing magical or mysterious in all of this. It is simply the intelligent organization of matter so that it is animated when it is created, and the combination of two bits of organized matter during reproduction.

Contemporary scientific research continues to contribute to the demystification of life, such as the young girl born in England who was conceived in a laboratory through the artificial combination of sperm and egg, and the re- implantation of these into a surrogate mother's womb. It is not surprising that this successful experiment was hotly condemned by the Catholic authorities, since it contributes to the removal of the 'mystery' of the creation of life, the 'mystery' upon which the church built its empire. There are many more experiments in progress which will demystify things completely. For example, one could quote the cloning experiments where a living being is created just from the genetic code taken from a cell of another being which is still alive. An American millionaire has already had a child which was produced purely from one of his own cells without the female element modifying his genetic code.

As a summary, and to make it more easily understandable for those who have done a bit of gardening, we can use an analogy, where the technique of cloning can be compared to growing a new plant from a cutting. Natural reproduction is like sowing seeds, and the creation of a new species by modifying an already existing variety's genetic code can be compared to creating a new hybrid fruit through grafting.

However the creation of a new species using only the basic chemicals cannot be compared to anything in this plant analogy.

So to complete this chapter, it is also important to demystify a concept which if not clarified could leave a dark shadow blocking the process of your awakening. The concept is 'love', which one might consider to be an exclusively human privilege, finally affirming our superiority over machines.

In fact this is not the case at all! We can just as easily programme a computer to love.

But first let us demystify this word 'love', behind which lie many different concepts.

Firstly, if that which you mean by 'love' is that which motivates two people of complementary sex to be nice to each other, with the ultimate goal being to couple with each other, then you need only look at birds for example, and their nuptial dances, to realize that animals do this far more artistically than most humans.

If what we mean by love is the sexual act itself, then the comparison is even easier. Remember that when we design an animal, we equip its sexual organs with nerve endings which make the love making more pleasurable. So by enjoying the pleasure that it procures, reproduction is assured in the animal, without it knowing it.

We have already seen that it is very easy to conceive of a computer able to build other computers, that is to say, capable of reproducing itself. We could just as well design these computers to be 'sexed', so that each one carries a half- plan necessary for the fabrication of another computer, which means that two complementary half-plans from two complementary computers must come together to make 'babies.'

We could easily have one computer which we could call 'male', designed to give its half-plan to the other and this other which we could call 'female' would combine the male's half-plan with hers to build the new computer which we would call the 'child'.

Whilst we are on the subject, it would be useful also to demystify the concept of 'pleasure'. While we could easily programme both computers to 'couple' their respective half- plans in order to re-produce a new computer in their image, for them to 'go forth and multiply', we would have to build in them organs which gave them pleasure as they transmitted their half-plans, thus ensuring that they will do it as often as possible.

What is pleasure?

Most recently, scientists have located pleasure centres in the brain. They have even been able to stimulate these areas with electrodes and the 'guinea pig subject' reported that he was feeling sensations similar to an orgasm. They were also able to prove that it was always these centres which were stimulated when someone was experiencing any sort of pleasure, (such as sexual enjoyment, a military person receiving a medal, a scientist or athlete receiving a reward or a caress etc)...

Now we know all about this pleasure centre and the process which allows us to feel any sort of pleasure. In fact, it is simply physio-chemical reactions occurring within the brain which produce electrical discharges experienced as pleasurable.

In the same way, other physio-chemical reactions can result in unpleasant sensations. The brain has been programmed to react in this way to certain exterior events and stimuli. This is what controls our behaviour. We seek things which give pleasure and avoid those which give pain.

So as to understand this phenomenon clearly, let us go back to the robot which returns to the mains socket to recharge its exhausted batteries. Let us imagine a simple needle on a dial indicating the amount of electricity remaining in the battery accumulator.

Beside this dial is another one showing the quantity of electricity entering the robot's rechargeable batteries when it plugs itself into the mains.

When the batteries are almost dead, the needle of the first dial goes almost to zero and triggers a contact relaying a signal to the computer, which is the robot's brain, informing it that it is time to go to the mains to recharge its batteries. This signal is disagreeable, just as hunger is disagreeable when it pains your stomach when it is soon time to eat after a day's fasting.

So our robot goes towards the mains and plugs in. Then the needle on the second dial is activated showing a maximum reading as it measures the amount of current entering. This triggers off another signal sent to the central computer which experiences it as pleasure, just like the first mouthfuls of a meal, or the first caresses before making love.

Gradually, the first needle which indicates the amount of accumulated current will go to the maximum reading, and when it reaches it, another contact will be made, triggering an electrical impulse informing the central computer that the batteries are now full. This impulse will be felt as a pleasurable satiety, in the same way that we feel a pleasurable satiety when our stomach is full after a good meal, or more explicitly, at the moment of sexual orgasm.

Then our robot unplugs itself and goes back to work just as we can do after a good meal or sexual relations. For to enjoy doing something, we must have abstained from doing it for a while beforehand, during which we do other things. As we will see later, it is the contrast between things which increase the sensation of pleasure, such as the contrast between hunger and eating, sexual abstinence and sexual activity, etc... We can thus see what the mechanism of pleasure is and consequently it is very easy to understand what love is when we are making love or preparing for it – it is physico-chemical reactions which trigger electrical impulses which the brain experiences as pleasurable and in no circumstances does it represent a superiority of man over machine since we can build a computer which can feel the same sensations.

Everything that we do, is done because it gives us pleasure, either directly or indirectly.

We eat because it gives us pleasure, we sleep, drink, make love, wash, groom ourselves... because it gives us pleasure. But we also pay our taxes because it indirectly gives us pleasure, ie, the pleasure of not going to prison. The woman who throws herself under a lorry's wheels to save her child, does it because it pleases her to do so. Otherwise she would not do it. The pleasure that she gets from saving her child is greater than the displeasure or pain that she would feel while being crushed by the lorry's wheels. The Japanese Kamikaze hurls himself and his plane at the enemy's ship because he gets more pleasure from the idea of dying for his country than displeasure at the thought of dying, otherwise he would not do it. Altruism is just another form of pleasure. Selfishness is another. But when we consider that the quality of pleasure that we get when giving pleasure to others is proportional to the number of people to whom we are giving pleasure, then altruism is a superior form of pleasure. What is more, the quality of pleasure is also proportional to what we consider the quality of the people to whom we are giving the pleasure. To satisfy a foolish crowd by giving them the pleasure of hearing what they want to hear, is far inferior to giving pleasure to one person if this person is wise or seeks to become wise. Between the rabble calling out for bread and distractions, and the person who is alone on the mountain to elevate his level of consciousness, it is to the latter that we must choose to give pleasure if we wish to elevate ourselves.

Even the person who dedicates his life to Humanity, does it because it is pleasurable and the reason why I am writing these lines is because it gives me pleasure to pass on to you the teachings which were given to me.

Thus we can see that even if we included what we call 'noble' sentiments behind the word 'love' such as altruism or devotion, though they may be nothing to do with sex, they are still based on the pleasure which they provoke in those who carry them out.

So it would be very easy to programme our robot so that it is able to put the interests of its child, companion, group or species above its own life. It is just a matter of needles and dials...

And so we have shown that even love for others doesn't represent a superiority of man over machine.

To conclude, what every concept we attribute or 'hide behind' the word 'love', it cannot be called a privilege only of Man, since love is mechanically reproducible.

Finally, one more word on the human ability to put ourselves in harmony with the Infinite which makes us up and which we are a part of. Even this ability cannot be called a superiority of man over machine. It would be very easy to conceive of a computer programmed to be aware of infinity, capable of feeling the infinitely big and infinitely small through the sensors which we have already mentioned, so that it can 'feel where it is at' and harmonize the energies which animate it.

This computer would be able to meditate with its senses, just as we are going to do, ie, practising Sensual Meditation.

Yet another non-superiority over machines!

Incidentally, the etymology of 'meditate' comes from the Latin 'meditare', which means to exercise. To exercise one's senses, that is the aim of Sensual Meditation.

Sexual differentiation

When using the example of the male and female robots, where the former gives his half-plan to the latter, who needs both plans to make a child robot, those who find it difficult to admit that we are not superior to machines could hide behind the question as to why some children turn out to be male while others are female.

We already know that in humans 'his' or 'her' sex is defined by the spermatozoon, that is to say the half-plan coming from the male, and nowadays, during artificial insemination, we know very well how to choose which sex we wish our child to be, since male and female spermatozoa are very easy to differentiate and separate.

So when a man transmits his sperm to a woman, if it is a male spermatozoon which combines with the woman's half- plan (the ovule), then the child who is born will be a boy, and if it was a female spermatozoon, then a little girl will see the light of day in nine months' time.

And so it is exactly the same with our robots who are capable of reproducing themselves. The robot which we will call a female robot, who will build another robot called the child robot, must have a complete plan (blueprint) to be able to build it. But she has only a half-plan which she must combine with another half-plan given to her by the male robot. It is the male's half-plan which will determine the sex of the child about to be built. When the male robot 'couples' with the female robot to give her the half-plan, in fact he gives her a large number of them, half of which are male half- plans, the other half, female half-plans. Only one will end up combining with the female's half-plan and it will be the one which chance put in the right place at the right time which will do it, in exactly the same way that only one spermatozoon among millions will manage to combine with the ovule during human conception.

4

VOLUNTARY DEPROGRAMMING

Every reaction and all our behaviour is due to the programming which we underwent throughout our education.

From the moment we were born, we have been unwittingly fashioned by our environment, parents, friends, educators, newspapers, films, etc... all have conditioned us to make us what we are today.

The way we sleep, wash, eat, dress, talk, walk, and even the way we judge others, everything, absolutely every part of our behaviour, is due to this unconscious conditioning to which we have been subjected.

Here again, to understand this phenomenon clearly, we must compare ourselves to a computer. The latter does only what it is programmed to do and has in its memory only what was put in it. It is just like us, the only difference being that we are capable of becoming aware of our programming, of analyzing the elements and of eliminating those which seem stupid in order to replace them with others. That is why we are computers capable of programming ourselves, therefore auto programmable.

The problem is that we have been programmed not only according to our own tastes, but by people who simply pass on and instill in us the same elements which were imposed on them without themselves having questioned them. For thousands of years, Man has been transmitting in this way, from generation to generation; a mode of conditioning, which through time became loaded with superstitions, fears and mysticism characteristic of all primitive societies.

The first stage of awakening consists of a re-questioning and re-evaluation of all our behaviour, and I mean all, from the way we eat to our own way of walking, including every reaction that we are in the habit of having in whatever circumstances, however harmless and insignificant they might seem to us.

The way we dress, to take an example, is not universal. We could just as well have been born in North Africa and worn a djellaba, or in the bush and worn a piece of cloth. Though the latter might not quite correspond to the requirements of our climate, the former certainly could. But for our parents, men wore shirts and trousers, and we wear the same thing as them, even though there is no objective reason to do so.

The same goes for the way we eat. Had we been born in China, we would be eating with chopsticks, and in certain parts of Africa, with our fingers. The use of the fork was not our choice, it was imposed upon us by our educators, even though it was not necessarily the best way. Take Chinese cooking for example, where food is served already chopped into small pieces, thus removing the need for a knife. Yet we (in the West) go on regardless with our custom of dishing out food which everyone must laboriously cut up on their own plate.

In this way, consider every act which you carry out during one day, and analyze it objectively, asking yourself precisely why you acted thus. You will be surprised to discover that there will be very few of them, maybe none for some people, which you did consciously, choosing to differ from what your parents do.

Admittedly, not everything taught to us during our education is bad, and certain elements can be kept as they are, but the important thing is to realize what is behind everything that we do.

The operation becomes more delicate when we start analyzing our reactions to actions and personalities of others. While it might be amusing (for a Westerner) to eat with chopsticks or wear a djellaba because of their exotic aspect, it becomes infinitely harder, once we have been conditioned to hate Arabs or make fun of homo-sexuals, to seek to understand them so as to accept them as they are.

How many times in our lives have we heard Arabs being talked of badly by people who consider them an inferior race, just because our ancestors dominated them with violence? So many times, that one day we even ended up repeating it. How many times have we heard of homosexuals being described as abnormal or perverted by people so ill at ease with their own selves, that they were afraid that these differences might uncover similar tendencies long buried within themselves? So often, that we ended up by saying the same stupid things ourselves.

The awakened person enriches himself through contact with the differences which constitute the personality of others. The closed minded person atrophies his brain by fighting these differences. And even as he dumbly insults them by using the same old clichés that, unknown to him, he was inculcated with, he would not be able to remove these differences.

The point is therefore to extract and sort out all the ideas which we received from those who shaped us. 'This one seems good for such-and-such a reason, therefore I keep it – that one seems bad, I eliminate it.' The criteria for choosing which ideas to conserve must depend upon what we think after having informed ourselves about them, rather than what our educators' opinions were.

This would be useless if one said merely: 'This idea must be good since my parents thought like that' – in fact, we should regard any of our ideas which are identical to those of our parents with complete suspicion.

Whether we are talking about Arabs or homosexuals, we should first meet one of them without any preconceptions, open oursel-ves to them and try to understand their reasoning, and then, only having done this, can we make up our own minds, being careful not to generalize from the personal characteristics of what may be the only subject whom we met, but basing our judgement only on the general points of the discussion.

But where this self questioning is essential in the hope of elevating our level of consciousness is in the area which concerns our sexuality and our conception of love.

LOVE OR SELFISHNESS

We have been continually impressed with a conception of love which implies definite and absolute possession and which has been bequeathed to us by thousands of years of fear and anguish. In the past, one would attack a village to acquire their gold, their horses, and... their women. All these things were considered to be goods capable of being exchanged and bartered without the slightest scruple.

After having recognized that if 'man' had a soul, then 'woman' must have one too (the Church doubted it for quite a time), after having granted them the right to vote (barely a century ago, and still not everywhere), we still do not recognize women's right to do freely with their body as they wish, by refusing them the right not to give life even if they do not want to (condemnation of abortion and contraception by the Church and certain governments).

What is more, if we kill someone whom we do not love, in order to steal their money, we can be condemned to life imprisonment, even death; but if we were to kill someone whom we claim to 'love' – what is called a 'crime of passion' – we can sometimes get off with only five or six years in prison! This means that we are living in a society which is encouraging its members to kill those they love.

The simple fact of conceiving that one can kill someone that one claims to love proves that we have quite a peculiar idea of love. Those who think in this way are in fact con- fusing love and selfishness, two things which are, however, very different and incompatible. In fact, the one who really loves someone thinks only of giving, but he who loves himself, and who is therefore selfish, thinks only of taking.

The selfish person is afraid that his partner might get more pleasure with someone else and abandon him, which will deprive him of the pleasure which he is in the habit of receiving, because what is important above all for him, is his personal pleasure.

The one who truly loves, hopes that his partner might meet someone who will give her even more pleasure, since what is important above all for him is the happiness of the other.

The selfish person watches over his partner so that she won't risk meeting someone else who will give her pleasure.

The one who truly loves, tries to facilitate his partner's contacts with other people who correspond to her tastes. When the partners of the selfish people meet someone who gives them pleasure, they will feel that they are stealing this happiness and will find it even better as forbidden fruit, which will bind them even more to their accomplices.

When the partners who are truly loved meet someone else who gives them pleasure, they will be grateful to their usual partner who had encouraged them to live these marvellous moments with someone else, and in most cases, they will both be enriched by this new experience.

And if the other really meets someone who fulfils them even more, then the one who truly loves will be filled with happiness at the thought that the one he loves is even happier than before, even if it is with someone else.

The selfish person prefers to keep 'his property,' he prefers his companion to be unhappy with him rather than happy elsewhere. And if that happens, he takes his gun to kill his 'loved one'... because he prefers that the one he claims to love is dead rather than happy with another. He does not see his partner's happiness, he only sees the pleasure that a stranger will take from the body of someone who belongs to him. It is exactly the same as a dog, who though not hungry, will not tolerate another dog approaching his bone. He'll bare his teeth and bury his goods just like the selfish person, since for the latter, his partner belongs to him, just as the dog owns the bone. All that counts is the pleasure that it gives him, and he prefers to remove it than see someone else benefiting from it. But so as to better understand the process which leads to the curse that is jealousy, which is but a form of selfishness, let us return to our auto-reprogrammable robots.

We saw that it was very easy to create a strain of 'sexed' robots, each possessing half a plan so that while 'coupling' they would create one complete plan and so allow the 'female' to make a 'child'. We also saw that to incite our robots to reproduce, we needed to render the act of coupling very pleasurable, so by equipping their sexual organs designed to transmit and receive their half-plans with nerve endings, the meeting of the two would generate pleasure.

When a 'male' robot meets a 'female' robot for the first time, they get to know each other, that is to say, they mutually discover a part of each other's programme and if they get on, that is to say, if their programming leads them to a certain 'spiritual' harmony, then they can let themselves satisfy the sexual desire building up in them, and connect.

They may then decide to live together so as to benefit as often as possible from the pleasure which they feel when united.

Then, one day, one of our robots might meet another robot whose apparent programming, whose 'charm' or... whose bodywork will strongly attract it. It is at that point that the habitual companion of our machine will have the choice between two forms of behaviour – it could seek the enrichment of its partner's programming with another and even encourage it, or it could prohibit all contact with other robots of complementary sex.

If it behaves in the second way, it can only be because it was programmed to behave in this way, since otherwise it could not consider itself to be the owner of another entity completely separate from its own body.

How can a person who meets another among the billions populating our planet suddenly say to himself 'here is the only individual with whom I shall henceforth have intimate relations, and even if I meet others who appear to correspond to my tastes, I shall stay faithful to the first, for the one and only reason that luck had it that they were there first.' That, in a nutshell, is 'fidelity'.

In fact, it is a striking observation that in many countries still undergoing the consequences of primitive civilization, women are still considered as merchandise to be bought. In the West, it's the father who provides the dowry for his daughter to find a spouse, who is often already interested in marrying her, whereas in the primitive societies, it is the husband-to-be who must offer the father of the young woman farm animals or other such presents.

This mixing between commerce and human relationships is scandalous. Potentially it can generate feelings of ownership which can lead to slavery. If it is tempting to consider someone whom one has just met as one's property, purely because one has become used to their presence, then it is even more likely to be so if one has 'paid' for such a companion.

Awakened people not only do not fear losing their partners, by encouraging them to live out all the experiences which tempt them, but on the contrary, they find themselves enriched by this and become even closer, especially as their sensitivity develops by the contact with people of differing personalities.

There also, contrast is a factor in the awakening process.

All this does not mean that you must force yourself to change partners in order to have a good chance of awakening yourself. One can be just as likely to have the good luck of having a companion who always knows how to be different while still being the same person, and who knows how to bring imagination and fantasy into the relationship which is indispensable to escape from habit, which is love's mortal enemy.

Thus the blossoming of each partner can continue in a permanent exchange of information, allowing each to benefit from the reflections and discoveries of the other and mutually developing their sensuality and consequently their level of awareness.

But though one must not force oneself to have experiences with others which one could live more intensely with one's partner, the whole, the composite organism which one forms with the latter must be an entity totally open to the exterior, that is to say, permanently ready for intimate contact with a third party. Each must understand that the enrichment of the other will enrich themselves.

Awakening is the permanent development of one's ability to communicate with one's environment and one's capacity for analyzing and integrating (linking) the information transmitted to us by our senses.

In fact the word 'intelligence' etymologically means just that, since it comes from the Latin 'intelligere' meaning 'interlinking of things', 'ligere' meaning 'to link'. Awakening is therefore a development of one's intelligence and one's capacity to understand, to comprehend; the word 'comprehend' being derived from the Latin 'comprehendere' meaning 'to bring together'.

It is also interesting to note that the word 'consciousness' comes from the Latin 'consciencia' which means 'know together.' Thus by elevating our level of consciousness, we raise our understanding and knowledge of the Infinite which is within us and which surrounds us.

This elevation allows the infinitely small within us and the infinitely large of which we are part, to 'know itself together' within us.

How Habits Atrophy Us

Habit, on the other hand, progressively atrophies the mechanisms for perceiving events. When we have just moved into a new flat and walk down the street for the first time, we notice everything, windows, colours, music, people we cross in the street, everything seems interesting. After a few days, we begin to perceive much less of the neighbourhood's atmosphere and our mind is filled more with our own personal introspections as we make our way to work. Then, with time, we may end up moving like a sleepwalker, perceiving almost nothing of our environment. We could almost go home reading the paper. That is habit. And when we behave like this with a partner, we progressively atrophy our capacity to communicate with our surroundings and diminish our intelligence.

The person whom we met, and whose appearance grabbed us by the feeling that it gave out, whose voice we found so charming, whose fragrance so intoxicating, now we live in their presence without even being aware of their existence. By repeatedly eating the same things in the same way, wearing the same clothes, making love at the same time, in the same position, we act mechanically, and allow the quality of pleasure obtained by our actions to become increasingly reduced, whereas it would hardly need anything, (it would take only a tiny bit of extra effort) to begin to re- discover the pleasure of marvelling at the life we lead and at each instant which passes, which we will never be able to live again.

It is in fact striking to observe that the progressive disintegration of faculties of an individual who allows himself to be invaded by habit is exactly comparable to the gradual decrease in enthusiasm of a population who allowed themselves to be choked by tradition.

This is why, if we wish to reach a maximum awakening of our faculties, we must live a life of maximum contrasts.

Not only visual, auditory, tactile, olfactory and gustatory contrasts, but also sexual and intellectual contrasts; basically in all ways of being, so as to make our life a totally original work of art, full of imagination and fantasy. Bear in mind that etymologically speaking, the Greek word 'phantasia' means 'apparition' and 'imagination', with imagination obviously being the apparition of images in the brain which are wilfully produced by the combination of known but previously unconnected elements which become linked by the intelligence (inter-ligere).

But so that these contrasts produce the desired effects, we must ensure that every one of the successive elements which come together to form these effects must be experienced as intensely as possible and that we miss none out. That is why every moment in our life must be lived to the fullest. We must 'grab the moment' as the poet would say, and 'the poet is always right because he sees beyond the horizon', ('le poete a toujours raison qui voit plus haut que l'horizon').

We must live every second as if it were our last with all the cells of our body, especially those which make up our receptors, through which we are aware of our surroundings. It is striking to realize, that when a loved one dies, we think back to the moments that we lived out with them, and regret not having given them more love or shown how much we loved them. Only death gives us this awareness, allowing us to realize how this negligence is irreparable.

The poorer one's level of awareness, the more he despairs at the death of a loved one. That is because he did not live those moments passed together intensely enough and he suddenly realizes that it is too late to do so now.

On the other hand, an awakened person does not grieve at the death of someone close, since he knows that he fully appreciated every second shared with that person, that he gave all the love that he could give, and that there was nothing more that he could have done to make him or her happier.

We also feel this intense emotion when someone whom we are fond of departs on a journey. In fact, it is often said that 'leaving is a little death' and this is because one is aware at that moment that our loved one could easily disappear en- route and one might never see him or her again. Therefore we seize that instant as we wave goodbye to him or her, appreciating it fully, and are full of regrets for not having also intensely lived all the moments during the days spent in their company.

It is also interesting to note that certain reactions of jealousy are caused by the lack of awareness of time passing when with a loved one. In fact, when our partner announces that he or she wishes to leave us, we suddenly think back to the times when we could have given a lot more love, but which we neglected and let pass without living intensely. So we then wish to start all over again and try to behave better, but after beautiful promises, we fall back into routine and habit until separation becomes inevitable. We experience this separation as a failure because it shows up our inability to live as we wish and be aware constantly of our actions so as to give the maximum amount of pleasure to this person we love. And yet, if we lived out every moment really intensely, all this would be possible, and all this not in order to keep the other person with us, but simply for the pleasure of not losing even one instant passing us.

Seizing The Moment

In fact one cannot live every moment intensely for any reason other than for the pleasure of living each moment intensely.

That is why the awakened person accepts separations with joy, since he knows that at every moment he gave the best of himself, that he enjoyed thoroughly the essence of every second and that he will fully enjoy the minutes yet to come during the separations. These separations will themselves be enriched by the memories of someone to whose awakening he contributed and whose harmony will in turn bring benefit to others.

The world we live in is responsible for a lowering of the level of consciousness, especially as far as time perception is concerned. We reach adolescence without even having realized that our childhood has gone by, then we find ourselves married with children ourselves and we didn't even notice our adolescence, then we discover ourselves old, without having noticed our lives going by. And we still feel that we haven't done what we wanted to do, or enjoyed fully the satisfaction of each age. We become shadowed by solitude and despair, and begin to hate the young, thinking that they know happiness which we've never had.

Thus back to jealousy again, where all that is needed to break this uninterrupted cycle which leads us like sheep from womb to tomb is a few moments of pause, so as to live the passing of time in a different way.

We jump from one action to another, without appreciating fully any of them, in a sort of constant flight forwards where we look forward constantly to what we are going to do, without being conscious of what we are doing right now. With joy, we imagine what we are going to do in the evening after work, but when we get back home, we switch on the television and since the programme is pretty mediocre, we watch it while looking forward to tomorrow's programme. And the next day, we do it all over again. The same goes for our annual holidays, we always think next year's will be better, but when we are actually there, we say 'it was better last year' and we start thinking about next year's ones...

When our partner is expecting a child, we imagine it playing with us and asking us questions, but when it is old enough to do so, we tell it to shut up and go to bed. Until one fine day, we realize that we are old without having had the time to live out the moments which have definitely passed.

And yet it is so easy to stop unconsciously letting events fly past us and learn to enjoy them fully, one needs simply to open one's eyes, one's ears and all one's senses and to pay attention to what is around us. We need to become aware mentally of our position in time, realizing how all the events in time made us what we are and put us where we are.

This mental re-situation in time must be carried out by reliving all the events of our existence which marked us, as far back through our childhood as we can go, remembering the faces, the voices and the smells of those who knew us when we were small, re-living those scenes which remain engraved somewhere in our neurons, up to the present time, including the teachers who influenced us, our first contacts, our first flirts, or our first job, etc. In this way, we will rediscover progressively the path which made us what we are, we will find the common thread linking all the events which moulded us to make the individual which we know today.

Once we have done that, we will need to see if the life that we lead is the one which we enjoy living and if that is not the case, then we must fix ourselves objectives so that it does become what we wish.

Having made this link with our past and what we wish our future to be, all that needs to be done is to live every instant with intensity, bearing in mind that it may be the last.

To live an event fully, one needs to be aware at the very moment that one is experiencing it, of the joy that one had when looking forward to it and to the pleasure that one will have when recalling it.

Someone said 'the best moment of love is when one is climbing up the staircase.' This is true for mediocre people. For the action itself to bring us even more pleasure than did expecting it or re-membering it, we must be conscious while carrying out this action, of the joy which we felt when going up the stairs and the memory that one would keep of the occasion afterwards.

What is more, this technique also allows us to obtain a better memorization of the event, which will enable us, simply by thin-king about it, to re-live it with an intensity almost as great as when it first occurred.

Finally, it is not possible not to mention masturbation while still on this fundamental subject of sexuality and its role in the awakening and fulfilment of the individual.

Masturbation – An Indispensable Stage

By stopping people from discovering the pleasures of self eroticism that their bodies give them, or by inflicting them with guilt at the highest level and associating touching oneself with evil, calling it unnatural and even dangerous or, as has been done for some time now, by telling those who indulge that it could make them blind, mad or paralysed, by doing any of these things, one is reducing the capacities of thousands of young people.

Those who dare tell such things to adolescents, who are entering a period of hyper-sensitivity due to major physical and hormonal changes, are simply criminals. How many of their own children did they give life-long complexes to and turn them into maniacs, 'impotents' and 'frigids'?

Now that science has been able to demonstrate how masturbation not only does not present any of the dangers that the medieval oracles predicted of it, but also that it is indispensable for the harmonious development of an individual during the critical period when one discovers one's own body, it is time to denounce out loud all those, including the Church first and foremost, who peddled such foolish and guilt inducing idiocies.

For adolescents, the act of discovering that, all of a sudden, their sexual organs give them enormous sensations of pleasure is fundamental to their development. A feeling of guilt created by their environment will in no way keep them from touching themselves, but instead they will continue to do so in a conflicted state of mind where the individual will begin to feel disgust toward their temptations, and as they unavoidably succumb, they will begin to feel disgust for their bodies, bearing the consequences for the rest of their lives. The most deeply unbalanced will be those rare cases who will be intimately convinced of the need for 'abstinence' from this self-eroticism known as masturbation, and who will abstain at huge cost and effort against themselves. This will make them harsh and cold individuals whose sensitivity will be reduced enormously, with all the consequences that this entails, both physically and mentally.

One must also add to this list of children seriously traumatized by being made to feel guilty of their natural reactions, all those who though they did not suffer such a treatment, were not informed by parents who were too afraid to face such a task and happy to say that 'one must not talk about anything touching upon sexuality or their organs.' More often than not, these parents themselves were badly informed and suffering from the sequels of a mystico-religious education seeing the body as bad and the mind as good.

However, all those who suffered such a guilt inducing education or who were lucky enough only to have to cope with the problem of awakening themselves, seeing as they could not rely on the illumination of their parents who were themselves too ashamed to even take the time to help their offspring understand what was happening to them, all those, and this is of special importance to the first lot whatever their age, can re-learn how to love the body and its reactions. They can re-learn to love their sexual organs and the pleasure which they can give them in all freedom and without the slightest feeling of guilt. What is more, they can re-live their so important discovery of self-eroticism, of which they had been deprived, and their adolescence in all awareness without all that they had previously suffered.

If this rebirth towards one's own sexuality is important for men, it is even more so for women, since as Betty Dodson says in her marvellous book 'The Feminine Orgasm', 'masturbation is the basis of sexual activity. Everything else that we do is no more than the socialization of our sexual life.' Among other things, through its excellently done illustrations, this book helps women to become aware of the beauty of their sexual organs which a male dominated society has always degraded and debased.

The first thing to do in order to re-live the adolescence which one has been deprived of, is to love one's body, even, and especially, the part which is able to give us the most pleasure and then learn how to discover and increase one's understanding of this organ so as to heighten the quality of joy that one can get from it.

The best way to understand fully how one's sexual organs work and to discover which caresses produce the strongest sensations of pleasure in the brain, is to experiment on oneself. No one can direct our fingers better than we can do ourselves so as to reach the exact spots which satisfy us most, and which differ for each individual anyway.

We can inform our partners of our specific tastes on the subject, so that they can do the things which we like, but to teach what we like to others, we must first teach it to ourselves.

While our sensuality is our link with Infinity surrounding us, self-eroticism is one of the most efficient ways to set off on the internal exploration of our computer. Self-eroticism is the lever which sparks off the physical reactions where men liberate their 'half-plans' and where for women, their organs become receptive for the meeting of the 'half-plans'.

It is also very important that those who live as a couple discover their capacities of self-eroticism together. In fact they could be even stronger precisely because of the presence of each other's bodies.

In this case too, the selfish mediocre person will not accept that his partner masturbates in his presence, since the person whose only use is to give him pleasure, is beginning to get pleasure by herself. What then is the use of his virility which he is so proud of and which he considers as his only unchallengeable superiority over women?

The selfish person is jealous even of the hand of his partner. The awakened person, on the contrary, rejoices at the sight of the person they love being happy and discovering her own profound mechanism of pleasure.

Once we have completed the destruction of ideas received concerning the basis of our sexuality, which is itself the roots of the tree of our personal blossoming, we can now think through once again in the same way, all our behaviour patterns, considering all the ways and all the subjects which make up our environment and which is our life.

By questioning everything which constitutes our personality, we are in fact carrying out a great spring cleaning and after having done this, we can go on to the next stage. However, we must bear in mind throughout our existence, that whenever we are faced with an issue which we have never thought about ourselves, we must proceed in the above way so that our reaction is a true reflection of our own thought.

Creating A Void

When the first day of self questioning and analysis of apparent personality has been completed, it is useful to practise the first exercise. This consists of creating a void in oneself and clearing out all the ideas which are jostling about within our minds and which create tensions most trying for our equilibrium.

One starts by sitting on the ground, either cross-legged or in any other position in which one finds comfortable, while breathing deeply for about 12 minutes and concentrating on one's breathing and nothing but one's breathing.

Then we concentrate on the fact that we are concentrating on nothing. The point is to clear out any idea appearing in our mind, whatever it might be, and with practice, manage to have no thoughts surfacing in our minds, not even the thought of not having any.

As we say earlier on, the brain is nothing more than a computer with electric currents running through it in all directions. This exercise is designed to balance these currents so as to obtain calmness and serenity. After practising this for a few minutes, we are then ready to act and think more efficiently. When seeking this absolute void, it is as important to cut oneself off totally from the outside world as it is from the inside one.

The aim is to try to become 'vegetable' for a few moments, in fact, even more vegetable than plants, since we know that plants can feel their environment. One could almost say that we are trying to become mineral.

No noise, no movement from anyone or anything, no odour and no sound is perceived by someone who is creating the void. This exercise is possible even in the middle of a crowd in a bustling street. In fact it is particularly useful for those living or working in a noisy environment.

In a way, we are putting ourselves into a state of sensory fasting. And this fasting, like all forms of positive abstinence, is designed to make us better appreciate the perception of what we were depriving ourselves of voluntarily. In fact, before embarking on the process of awakening, it is extremely useful to fast for a day, both sensorially and so far as food is concerned, just drinking a lot of water to purify our organism.

To manage keeping a permanently new state of mind, it is of capital importance to be aware that we never perform an action proper to ourselves, but all our actions are merely reactions to something else. The only action which we can decide upon personally, is not to have a reaction.

Everything that we do during our life which we think are actions are in fact no more than a succession of reactions.

The simplest fact of being born is no more than the react- ion to the mating of our parents which occurred nine months beforehand. Then we cried because we were hungry and we were hungry because we burned energy through living, etc... Now you are reading this book, and that is due only to an advertisement or an interest in the subject. An interest in a subject which was only a reaction following the education given to you, or a reaction against this education. In this way, we can trace back all our reactions to our birth, then to that of our parents, going right back to the first humans who were created. And they themselves were created only as a reaction of our creators who had reached a level of scientific know- ledge allowing them the wish to do such an experiment. And these creators themselves lived only as a succession of reactions, etc. We could continue this train of thought, which is only a reaction, indefinitely. In fact, that would contribute to us becoming aware of infinity.

As for myself, I am transmitting this teaching as a reaction to the meeting with the extra-terrestrials who asked me to do so and who are guiding us.

Thus it is, when we become aware of the infinite series of reactions that we have had ever since we existed, and which we thought were actions, that we must understand the importance of always being conscious of the reactions which we chose to have.

When people jostle us in the street or insult us, they expect us to have certain reactions which they might hope for if they wish to fight us. If we react with further insults, we are providing just those reactions which they are waiting for, so that they can then become violent. If on the other hand, we refuse to react to their insults and continue on our way, thus refusing to give a reaction, we have then performed our own action, proper to our own self.

When we are doing the exercise where we create the void, refusing all reaction to our environment as well as to our thoughts, we are entering a situation where our action becomes proper to ourselves.

The person who initiates this process, escapes the uninterrupted cycle of unconscious successive reactions and consequently begins to elevate his level of consciousness.

5

VOLUNTARY REPROGRAMMING

Discovering Our Own True Tastes

After having voluntarily deprogrammed ourselves and having cleared out our minds by doing the void, we can now awaken our whole being to our immediate environment and then to the infinity which encompasses us, through that which links us to all this, our senses.

'They have eyes, but they do not see, they have ears, but they do not hear', such is a description of the people who surround us and who we resembled before we became aware of ourselves.

In exactly the same way that when a baby is born, it progressively discovers the world in which it is cast, through the sense of touch, taste, smell, hearing, and sight, so too shall we be reborn through our senses to all that surrounds us except that this time we shall be totally aware of the process. The act of developing our sensuality will allow us to discover the things that deep down we really don't like, even though in the past, we thought that we liked them because we accepted and became used to them through our conditioning. By the same token, it will also allow us to discover that there are many other things that deep down we really like even though we thought that we hated them because our education did not give us the opportunity to try them out.

The functioning of our senses is based on the perception of contrasts, such as contrasts in temperature or roughness for the sense of touch, in flavours for the sense of taste, in fragrances for the sense of smell, and in shapes and colours for vision.

To develop our sensuality means to develop our ability to perceive changes through our senses, especially the effects that these produce in us.

The mediocre person perceives only the large differences existing in the food that he swallows at great speed, and besides that, his taste buds have also deteriorated through alcohol, tobacco or stimulants. For him, it is totally incomprehensible that one could taste a difference in two types of water. If you are in this category, do not worry, for once you have given up smoking, the sense of taste returns bit by bit, and after a few weeks begins to develop normally. This same mediocre person perceives differences in smells only when they are huge. For him, it either 'smells good' or it 'smells bad' and nothing else. Don't bother asking him if he noticed that his partner put roses in the lounge. Unless he saw them, he won't even realize that they are there.

For the sense of hearing, it is exactly the same, so long as there are drums and an electric guitar, then it is music. Grasping the subtleties of classical music or synthetic sounds is out of the question.

The same goes for sight, the colours on the television are set at a maximum so that the contrast will be as large as possible. No chance in him grasping the subtleties and colour ranges of a master-painting or spotting a flower in the middle of a field.

And finally for the sense of touch, this insensitive person, who unfortunately represents the majority of our contemporaries, does not know how to caress. He can hardly recognize hot from cold and is totally incapable of distinguishing the softness of two cloths. For him, to caress means to knead brutally and the only reason why contact with feminine skin is pleasurable is because it precedes a brutal and impersonal ejaculation which is accomplished from time to time, more often than not, only because it is a conjugal 'duty'.

Let us quickly forget this horrific description which, sadly, is that of the majority of present day 'humans', to look at how it could be otherwise and especially how to get there.

It is all based on an improvement in the perception of contrasts.

But before proceeding any further, it is most important to make the following point: no valid improvement of one's sensuality can be obtained by someone who smokes, even if it is just a few, or who drinks alcohol, or who takes excitants including tea and coffee, or obviously who does all these at the same time. It will be useless to try to refine one's perception of infinity while continuing to clog up one's perceptual organs. It is a bit like putting cotton-wool in your ears before going to listen to a concert.

Let us start with the sense of touch. To improve our tactile perception means to improve our capacity to differentiate between the temperatures and textures of things that we are touching, by becoming aware in an increasingly subtle way of the effects that they produce in our brain.

We start with the things that contain the largest differences and then we whittle down these differences until we have great difficulty in perceiving them. Thus we define our degree of tactile sensitivity, and through exercises, we manage to refine the quality of perception while we ourselves will be witness to our own progress. When we caress something or someone, we must be totally at the tip of our fingers, so as to become what we are touching, and fit into the slightest contour, while all the time enjoying fully the effect that this has on us.

The way to start developing the sense of taste will be

exactly the same, this time taking time to analyze the flavours of what we are eating, and even what we are drinking, especially water. When you are tasting, become the taste buds and follow the path taken by this chemical message to your brain and the way it decodes it. To develop one sense, you must short circuit the others completely, so as to mobilize your consciousness on the one with which you are concerned.

If the blind have a highly developed sense of touch, hearing and smell, it is because they compensate for the absence of their visual perception by improving the quality of their other receptors.

To develop one sense is to pretend to be 'blind' in all the others, whilst we exercise one intensely.

We are linked to infinity which surrounds us through our senses and only through our senses. A person who cannot touch, taste, smell, hear or see, will be totally unconscious. Consciousness is developed through sensuality.

We cannot conceive of infinity, we can only feel it.

It is these exchanges which are produced in us, between our organism and the Infinite within which we evolve, which makes us alive. The ordinary man is made up of these interchanges but is not aware of them, which creates imbalances within him causing physical or mental illnesses, resulting in aggression or violence.

The awakened person is aware of these exchanges and improves them, which allows him to be in harmony with himself and Infinity at all times.

What is more serious, is that the ordinary man sometimes hinders these exchanges or atrophies willingly them to obey guilt-inducing precepts which were handed on to him by generations of violent and warlike people who gave rise to the world which we know today and which accumulated the weapons of its own destruction.

The awakened person develops these interchanges to the maximum and becomes the Earth when stroking a rock, a cherry tree when eating a cherry, a rose when smelling a rose, a nightingale when listening to one sing and a universe when contemplating a star-filled sky.

The mediocre person feels alone and isolated, cut off from everything and cuts himself off from everything through a fear of contact, due to a lack of awareness and to the progressive atrophy of his physical means of communicating with his environment.

The awakened person feels linked to everything, and makes love with every molecule of his body and to every star in the sky. The sense of smell too, must also be developed progressively, by an increasing perception of contrasts which must be preceded by a period of purification for those who were smokers.

The sense of hearing must also be allowed to recover if you have taken up the habit of frequenting 'nightclubs' or 'rock- concerts' where the volume is so loud that, according to a serious study, all those who frequent them are 30 per cent deaf. That means that at least one quarter of our auditory capacity, that is to say, one quarter of the possible amount of communication with Infinity, is missing for millions of young people! All we need to do is to impose upon ourselves a period of auditory abstinence during which we must be careful to avoid all sound and all music. Bit by bit our auditory organs will regain all their sensitivity and we can rediscover the sounds of our environment and music with all its richness at a normal level.

Finally, our sight must be refined in its capacity to perceive the subtle nuances in colour and to convey the stimuli which condition our state of mind. We know that red is exciting and green is calming, for example, but every tint has properties which we can discover by improving our visual perception.

Once the five senses begin to be developed sufficiently, then we can practise within ourselves the mechanisms of synesthesia. We can thus see a colour by listening to a sound, hear a sound by smelling a fragrance or have a taste in our mouth by looking at a colour.

This sublime feast of the senses opens up one of the most important doors of our minds, by producing in us one of the effects that drugs have and which the youth of the entire world is seeking. These can be obtained without the slightest degree of danger, through the natural mechanisms which practice in Sensual Meditation provides, by improving our sensuality and therefore by making us aware of what links us with Infinity.

'Perfumes, colours and sounds all answer each other,' said Baudelaire, who had synesthesia without knowing it. Let us be bathed in the harmony of all these sensations, let us be enveloped by all the perceptions of Infinity which mingle in us to fling us into a whirlwind of pleasure from which we will emerge yet stronger and more sensitive, to thus make of our planet a world of happiness by elevating the level of awareness of our peers, and allowing them to discover the treasure hidden in each of them.

6

PROGRAMME OF SENSUAL MEDITATION

The programme of Sensual Meditation is taught usually as a course of awakening which lasts for one week and contains a total of a dozen exercises. Following the fantastic results obtained by these techniques, and because a daily practice of Sensual Meditation is indispensable for reaping all the benefits, many people who followed the courses in France and Canada have manifested their desire to have them recorded on CDs and audio cassettes.

For this reason, six basic exercises were selected and recorded onto compact discs which can be obtained in any of the four centres of Sensual Meditation which were all opened simultaneously in Paris, Geneva, Brussels and Montreal.

In these centres it is also possible to come to meditate, alone or as a group. Teachers are waiting there for you, who will allow you to discover all the facets of these teachings, as well as other exercises which cannot be taught by CDs. Furthermore, some of these recordings are designed to be listened to when accompanied by a partner of complementary sex, and so those who are single can hope to meet another person in these centres with whom they can be sure to find spiritual harmony, since they are mutually interested in the same process of awakening and with whom they can also hope to find physical harmony.

These centres will also, among other things, allow those who might not have such an harmonious residence to come to spend a few hours whenever they like, in a place designed to satisfy their five senses through its decoration and layout. A place of teaching, where people who have chosen the same path for awakening can meet and a place of exchange where they can improve their sensory perception of Infinity, guided by teachers who take up any problems of all new arrivals as their own in order better to solve them; that is what is meant by a centre of Sensual Meditation.

Now we shall outline the six basic exercises which are recorded in the programme of Sensual Meditation.

Meditation 1 - Harmonization With Infinity

Ideally, this meditation should be practised outside, if possible under a starlit sky. But since the weather does not always bring together such favourable conditions, it might be preferable to kit yourselves out with a meditation room, harmoniously decorated with posters, paintings, sculptures or other works of art which you particularly enjoy. See to it that the lighting is soft or indirect, if possible with reddish tints or better still, use candlelight. This is for your visual sense.

You can burn some scents, as voluptuous as possible. This is for your second sense: smell.

Lay down a very soft surface for lying on, which is also pleasant to stroke, but don't make it too soft so that your body may be maintained quite straight when lying down on it. This is for your third sense, touch.

Try to have a good quality high fidelity sound system in order to get all the musical nuances. This is for your fourth sense, hearing.

For the fifth sense, taste, stimulate your mouth before starting, with a fragrance which you like (mint, aniseed, fruits, etc).

Make sure that the room temperature is sufficiently high for you to be naked without feeling cold (22 degrees Centigrade at least). Total nudity is ideal in order to feed your body fully, but wearing a meditation gown made out of a very soft and silky material can bring about further sensations by its contact.

A lukewarm and perfumed bath just before the meditation is an excellent preparation.

It is very important after coming home from work to take off the clothes which you worked in, which are often in disharmonious or polluted atmospheres, and to at least take a shower and put on this meditation robe, which could be either a djellaba or a gown, made from a material so soft and silky that you can enjoy being caressed through it. The colour of this piece of clothing should be your favourite one and if you do not have any preferences, white will do very well.

It is indispensable, especially for men, to be totally naked under this robe so that the male sexual organs, which are usually submitted to a genuine torture by today's fashion of tight trousers which is responsible, among other things, for a great number of cases of impotence, can regain their normal position, blood flow and temperature which is upset when they are compressed.

Now let us listen to the first CD or audio tape.

Lie down comfortably on the surface designed for this purpose so that your body weight is distributed equally. Place your hands along your body, palms facing upwards. It is essential to be in a comfortable position which you can keep up for a very long time without needing to move.

Then close your eyes and listen...

I
THE IMPORTANCE OF BREATHING

What is breathing? Why do we breathe? As you certainly know, we fill our lungs with fresh air rich in oxygen and then exhale air rich in carbon dioxide.

Our lungs are organs in which our blood eliminates carbon dioxide which it took from our cells and loads itself with oxygen which it will then bring to all the cells which form our body.

The majority of people breathe very badly. The simple fact of sometimes needing to sigh proves bad breathing. He who breathes well, never sighs.

A few moments of conscious breathing every day improves our health and accelerates the process of awakening.

We have seen how the brain is nothing other than a biological computer. Secretions of chemicals are being constantly produced in our brains which spark off electric discharges which form our thoughts and which are responsible for both the physical balance of our body as well as our mental equilibrium. If the latter is under-oxygenated, then these secretions are weak, or as a reaction to the lack of oxygen, become too abundant, which then give rise to all the imbalances which provoke physical and mental illnesses.

If our breathing is sufficient, then the oxygenation of the cells which make up this central computer which is our brain provokes an improvement of the chemical secretions within it and finally a harmony spreads throughout our whole organism. To be in harmony simply means having a brain which is functioning to its optimum in the management of the organism that it is controlling.

That is why you must commit yourself to a few minutes of breathing at the beginning of each exercise of Sensual Meditation and obtain an over-oxygenation of your body which will trigger an acceleration of the chemical exchanges within it, especially within our head.

It is vital to breathe very deeply for at least three minutes before each exercise; but the results will be far better if you have enough time to extend it to 12 minutes of oxygenation. It is also important during the exercise to be totally concentrated on our breathing and to be fully aware of the effects that this produces on our organism. By being conscious of this action, the effects are increased even more through a process of feedback.

II
Becoming Aware Of The Infinitely Small
Of Which We Are Composed

The second part of this first CD in the programme consists of becoming aware of the infinitely small of which we are composed. The aim is to connect together all the cells of which we are composed and which are all linked through nerves to the central computer which is our brain. In this way, these subtle unconscious interconnections must become conscious so that their quality might improve, enabling one to feel totally coherent and integrated, first physically and then mentally.

The first CD is the most important one of the Sensual Meditation programme since it constitutes the basis, the trunk of the tree of knowledge, which we shall see grow in us and of which the later exercises will only be the branches.

The point of this exercise is for the body to become aware of the cells which make it up and for the cells to become aware of the body which they compose. Each one of these building blocks called cells, of which we are made, feels suddenly linked directly with those immediately surrounding it and linked indirectly with all the others via the brain computer which links them all together.

Towards the end of the exercise, it is the computer itself which becomes aware of the matter that it is made of, with all these neurons which allow it to feel itself. It is matter becoming aware of both itself and its own awareness.

At that moment, our whole organism is so filled with waves of energy circulating in all directions between the brain and every cell, that we experience a sensation of well-being that even provokes crying in the more sensitive among us. You should certainly not fight the phenomenon, which is no more than a chemical reaction resulting from the well-being that the cells which compose us experience, when at last they feel connected and united totally with each other. On the contrary, you should enjoy fully this fabulous moment, rich in harmonious pulsations.

In fact, it was this which was the original meaning of the 'collect', (in French, the word is 'recueillement'), which is part of some religious ceremonies involving terrible minutes of silence, having totally lost its deeper physical significance. To 'collect' oneself comes from the Latin word 'colligere' which means 'to co-link' or 'to link together' and in this context means to link together that of which we are composed.

III
Becoming Aware of One's Level

At this point of the exercise, our whole 'collected' organism whose parts are united and integrated totally, will become aware of its surroundings purely through the sense of hearing, by listening to the music.

By becoming aware of the music through the intermediary of this sense, whose functioning is based on the perception of vibrations which we call sound, our body as a whole is then able to perceive these musical vibrations. As it listens to the music, our body is suddenly aware of something not coming from itself, which has an effect of accentuating the phenomenon where the cells become aware of their unity, and this gets the cells to vibrate in unison with an even greater feeling of solidarity among themselves, every one united totally in a rush of global harmony.

Finally, waves have the property of being made up of nothing while animating the medium in which they are travelling, and so the organism which listens not only with its ears but also with all the pores of its skin, becomes the music to which it listens, because it is penetrated and traversed throughout by the music's vibrations.

IV

Becoming Aware Of The Infinitely Large Of Which We Are A Part

Once the organism that is in harmony with itself and has become aware of its ability to get in harmony with what it can pick up from its environment, it can then try to get in harmony with the infinitely large, of which it is a tiny part. This is the aim of the penultimate phase of this CD and which opens up to us the movements which, though we might not be aware of it normally, shoot us through the infinite galaxies. Our Earth is spinning on its own axis while at the same time rotating around our sun, our sun is rotating around the centre of the galaxy, while our galaxy itself is moving around another point. As all these movements add up 'ad infinitum', we end up being hurtled through an infinite dance at unimaginable speeds, yet as we lie down on the ground, we usually tend to think that we are lying still... And somewhere above us in this cosmic immensity, there are some people watching us who love us as their own children. This way of looking at the infinitely large allows someone who is already in harmony with the infinitely small which composes him and who is capable of resonating fully to the rhythm of the surrounding waves, to become aware of the immense size of the universe in which he lives and the natural cosmic harmony of which he is a small part, and in which he is bathing permanently.

The act of feeling this harmony which exists in the infinitely large in which we are navigating, strengthens the integration which has settled in our constituents cells, through a process similar to mimicry. As our organism realizes suddenly that it is surrounded by harmony, it feels obliged to become harmonious itself.

V
REALISING HUMANITY'S POTENTIAL

The last part of this exercise consists of becoming aware of Humanity, of which we are an element; that is to say, returning to our level and opening ourselves up to how our planet could be if everyone were to vibrate together in the same total harmony which brings about fraternity and universal peace automatically.

The act of understanding that everyone can feel this fantastic well being, allows us to realize how we ourselves are cells of a huge body called Humanity and that we can take part in the spreading of this wave of love on a planetary level by sharing what we have felt with everyone around us, allowing all those who haven't yet had the good fortune of doing so to know the joy of discovering the natural harmony in which they are unconsciously bathing.

It is this exercise which allows us to feel 'high' the fastest and to feel, naturally and without danger, the sensations obtained normally through the use of drugs. There are many young drug users who have stopped using these dangerous substances after having discovered that they can 'trip out' far more powerfully, but without the terrible feelings of need, and what is more important, becoming at the same time even more efficient, in their professional and sexual lives.

Drugs produce altered states of consciousness by establishing certain 'short circuits' in the brain which, though these might produce pleasant sensations in the short term, actually damage the functioning of the brain. Sensual Meditation allows one to obtain the same sensations, but far stronger and more permanently, since instead of altering the state of consciousness through short circuits, it elevates the level of awareness by developing our natural mechanism, which through training will be able to function better and better as we use them more and more.

Drugs enable us to discover certain ecstatic experiences by atrophying the natural mechanisms which are designed to allow us to reach them, whereas Sensual Meditation develops these mechanisms, thus allowing us to reach these ecstasies more and more easily. The totally awakened person is able to live permanently in a state of absolute joy. To reach such a level of awareness may require many years of work upon oneself, usually seven years. For those who are already fairly awakened or who have already started to meditate, it will take far less time.

Meditation 2 - Becoming Aware Of Our Life Rhythms

To begin with, this second CD or tape will allow us to become aware of our breathing, but this time in a more physical way compared with the last exercise.

The point is to feel the whole of our respiratory apparatus by, after having held our breath, contrasting the feeling of fresh air which we breathe in with the residual warm air left in the lungs and bronchial tubes.

Our sensuality is developed by feeling contrasts, such as differences in temperature, colour, sound or odours.

After having oxygenated ourselves thoroughly, as we do before all of these exercises, we then tune into our lungs and live out this fantastic chemical exchange thanks to which we are alive – the oxygenation of our blood.

Then we concentrate on feeling our heart beat, this pump which passes the blood through our lungs so that it picks up

those precious oxygen atoms for which our whole body is waiting.

So as to feel our heart beating more easily, we can press lightly the tips of our right hand against those of our left.

By doing this, first we can feel this regular rhythm easily in the tips of our fingers, and then in the whole hand, and progressively we will try to feel it everywhere, in the arms, in the whole body and finally in the brain itself, where it feels as if we can hear the heart beat. Thus we become aware of our heart as we feel it beat calmly and harmoniously in our chest. Through other exercises taught at the course of awakening, we can learn how to slow down or speed up our heartbeat at will, just as we can choose to slow down or speed up our breathing, even though usually, as with the heart, its rhythm is regulated by the brain without us having to think about it. The first CD integrated our organism, whereas this one makes us aware of the rhythms which are animating and keeping it living continually. This allows us to feel alive,

pulsating right up to our finger tips to the best of this pumps ability, whose every action is essential and which is just as much 'us' as is the brain which is aware of it.

Meditation 3 - Body Awareness

Now that we have interconnected the cells forming our body and felt the rhythms which animate it, in this meditation we shall become aware of our body through our senses.

The first two exercises occurred within ourselves and consisted of our organism becoming aware of itself through totally internal mechanisms without requiring the use of our external senses.

Now we are going to discover our physique, first through our sense of touch, by keeping our eyes closed and then through each of the other senses.

Discovering our body through the sense of touch allows us to become aware of the sensitivity of different parts of our organism and to enjoy the pleasure of both being toucher and touched, stroker and stroked.

However, for the first few times that we do this exercise, we must try to be more in the tips of our fingers than in the rest of our body and be just the toucher so as to become aware of the shape and form of our body through our own hands. In this tactile exploration of our own shape, we rediscover the pleasure that we once had as babies when we explored ourselves, except that this time we are fully conscious of what we are doing.

The feelers are being felt themselves. This is particularly obvious when we start sucking the tips of our fingers to feel them better. At the same time, we are discovering the taste of our own skin. By sucking our fingers and then the skin of our own arm, we discover what we taste of, our own unique flavour.

Then, still with our eyes closed, we explore our own body smells. In fact it is important not to have taken a soapy shower just before this exercise, and obviously not to have put on any deodorants or perfumes. The best thing would be to take a soapy shower the evening before this exercise and then allow the body to produce overnight the secretions responsible for our body smells.

The next stage consists in discovering our voice by feeling oursel-ves talk, as much with our hands as with our ears. 'I am touching this head, which is me emitting sounds.' Thus we listen to ourselves as if we were someone else listening to another person speak.

Finally we open our eyes to discover ourselves through our sense of vision, first by looking at our hands moving, just as a baby does in its cot, except this time we are fully conscious of the beauty of our limbs and their movements.

Then we caress once again our body with our hands, discovering every part of our physique as if we were looking at it for the first time. It is very important to have a portable mirror beside us from the start of the exercise, to help us look at certain less-accessible parts of our body.

We look at ourselves as if with new eyes. We have never taken the time to look at certain parts of our body with love, particularly our sexual organs, because of the taboos passed on to us by our parents. This is especially true for women, whose sexual organs were considered 'dirty' by phallocratic societies.

Our sexual organs, which give us pleasure and which can give life, are as beautiful as flowers for both men and women. In fact, flowers are plant's sexual organs.

Our anus itself, which we can see using our mirror, is a magnificent part of our body. It is through there that matter is evacuated, matter which has been in contact with every part of the inside our body, that we can never touch, and which has left the best of itself so that we can live.

After having discovered with amazement this fabulous living toy, which is our body, and which expects only one thing, namely, that we enjoy it, we can then re-establish contact with our environment, where other people are developing and who like us, have just been able to become aware of these treasures of which we are composed and which we have ignored for far too long.

Meditation 4 - Meditation Facing The Symbol Of Infinity

The CD or tape should be listened to sitting down as comfortably as you can and, if possible, sitting cross-legged in contrast to the first three exercises which were to be done lying down.

The poster showing the symbol of Infinity which may be obtained along with the CDs should be stuck on a wall at eye level and if possible illuminated by a bright light, with the rest of the room in darkness. Once a person has tuned into himself and totally awakened to themselves internally through the previous exercises, he can then become aware of something entirely foreign to himself and allow himself to be invaded by the vibrations transmitted by the drawing's shape. Every shape around us is influencing permanently us and the most recent experiments using small pyramids have shown that fruit can be dehydrated completely without going bad purely as a result of waves reflected off walls angled and orientated in a certain way.

We also know that when sounds are analyzed electronically, 'O' produces an O form on the screen while 'I' shows an I form.

Every colour and sound emits specific vibrations which can harmonize with themselves and influence our behaviour and well-being, and in the same way, the waves of form produced by our environment exert an enormous influence upon our development and fulfilment.

As explained in the beginning of this book, this symbol represents Infinity in space and time and emits particularly harmonious waves of form. It is not by chance that it can be found in the Tibetan Book of the Dead, or dotted all over India in places well known for their traditional emphasis on the blossoming and development of the individual, even though it is now buried under years of superstition.

The 'watchmaker' left traces of how his watches function, particularly in this huge continent.

To get maximum benefit from this exercise, it is most important to understand that this symbol has absolutely nothing to do with the Nazi criminals who stole part of it for their emblem. In any dictionary a 'swastika' is described as 'religious symbol of India' (from the Sanskrit 'su' = well and 'asti' = being). At this moment there are millions of people meditating in their Buddhist temples decorated with this symbol, just as their ancestors have done daily for thousands of years. If Hitler had used the Christian cross as his symbol instead, (and he almost did since it would have helped him in his project of Jewish genocide) would that have meant that after the war Christians all over the world would not have been allowed to carry or use their symbol? Obviously not. In the same way, the fact that the Inquisition killed thousands of people in the name of the Christian cross does not reduce Jesus' message of love and fraternity.

It was important to write that paragraph since it is impossible to awaken ourselves and blossom while contemplating a symbol which we think is an emblem of violence. On the contrary, this combination of the two triangles interlocked into each other and the swastika, is the emblem of absolute love, infinity, life and joy.

The triangle pointing upwards represents the infinitely big, which includes the stars and galaxies swirling around us, or more precisely together with us, since we aren't the centre of the universe, not even that of our own solar system.

The triangle pointing downwards represents the infinitely small, including cells which compose us, which are themselves independent organisms as well as integrated with each other, molecules which make up our cells, atoms which are themselves universes containing planets upon which people like us live and who look up at their sky, wondering whether life exists elsewhere.

The stars of our sky make up our galaxy in which we bathe. Our galaxy is a part of our universe, which itself is a tiny bit of a huge particle situated somewhere in a cell in the body of a gigantic living being, which itself is contemplating its own sky, wondering whether there is life elsewhere.

The infinitely large is composed of the infinitely small and without the infinitely small there would be no infinitely large, which is why the two triangles are interlinked.

As for the swastika, it represents infinity in time. Every- thing around us has always existed, either in the form of matter, or in the form of energy. The matter of which we are made has always existed and will always exist because we are made of eternity. Only its form changes. We are but the organized accumulation of particles taken from the food which was absorbed by our mother, and which came together according to a specific plan to form us in her womb. Then after our birth these particles came from the food we ate, some from carrots, others from potatoes, meat and eggs, etc. But the carrot eaten by our mother or by us, of which an atom might have remained in our nose, for example, will have extracted this atom from the soil in which it grew. It came to this soil from the compost brought by the gardener, and before that was in the dung coming from a cow's intestines. Before that it was part of a mouse which, after being eaten and excreted by a carnivore, was absorbed by the grass which the cow ate, etc... In this way, we could follow the story of this particle which is in your nose right back to a time preceding the creation of life on Earth, and the same goes for all the particles of which you are made: they have always existed. Some have even been part of other people's bodies, living hundreds or thousands of years ago.

That is what the symbol which we are contemplating represents, and as we do so, it irradiates us with its beneficial vibrations.

The technique of looking at it as described by the CD is designed to imprint its image on our retina and especially to inform our computer of its exact shape. Prolonged exposure to these vibrations elevates our degree of harmony even more. This develops our ability to perceive Infinity through its vibrations in which we are bathing.

Meditation 5 - Discovering Another Universe : Our Partner

In contrast to the first four exercises, this one cannot be done alone, a partner is necessary. If we are with someone with whom we are thinking of making love, then this is an excellent preparation for the relationship to be a success; alternatively, if we have been having an intimate relationship already with someone for a long time and wish to rediscover each other and bring a new light to the relationship, where each awakens the other simultaneously, then this, too, is an excellent preparation.

However, this CD can also be listened to when we are with someone with whom we do not wish to have any sexual contact, but in whose company we simply wish to develop our personal awakening and blossoming.

The previous CD consisted of someone, already fully self- harmonious, opening themselves to the outside world and becoming aware of it through an inert symbol which was imprinting its waves of form into them.

Now this universe which we are, and which has become conscious of its own internal harmony, is going to discover another universe made in its own image by massaging gently its partner's whole body, who, once finished, will turn the cassette over and listen to it again, except this time, the one who was massaged now becomes the masseur: the discovered is now the discoverer. Thus two universes will have known each other mutually. The French word 'connaissance' means 'being born' or 'entering into the world together'. As we have seen, our body is a universe, and thus a world, and when we become aware of something around us it becomes part of our world and thus is born to us. When two people meet each other, they mutually enter into each other's world.

The massage is not supposed to be a form of physiotherapy, and to do it one need not have any prior knowledge of kinesitherapy. The aim is simply to become aware, through the sense of touch, of another person's shape and how they are a body of cells and atoms just like us, susceptible to the same reactions as we are.

Neither must it be erotic. We are not caressing, we are gently kneading the organism which we are discovering, steadily moving up towards the heart. It is better to press slightly too hard than too soft. We are becoming aware of the texture of our partner's flesh as we follow the contours of their bones through the skin. Our thumbs are working and kneading this living matter which makes up another world.

As for the one being massaged, this exercise produces even more important effects in us as we become aware of another anism through their hands. We were lying there in absolute harmony, when suddenly, something foreign to ourselves started to feel our body. The first reaction is a feeling of tension or a sort of coiling away from something alien. Then, bit by bit, our body realizes progressively that the effects produced by this contact are positive and marvellously relaxing, until the finger movements on our skin are expected, anticipated and wished for, particularly in those parts where the hands have not yet been and where you know that they will go.

This expectancy turns to pleasure and increases the feeling of unity of our whole organism.

When this CD is finished, we have reached the end of the part of the programme addressed to people without sexual partners, since the next exercise is designed for the moments preceding physical union of two people of complementary sex. The act of discovering that physical contact with others is possible without necessarily being sexual, is going to modify deeply our reactions towards others. We will not see those close to us and those we meet in the same way that we used to. This new vision of humans around us will multiply our capabilities for communication tenfold.

Henceforth we will no longer consider others as people with whom we can communicate only through sound and sight, as our medieval education taught us, now we can see them as living beings whom we can also touch and who can touch us if they have understood the importance of this contact and have accepted it so as to develop and blossom further.

It has been proven that children need this physical contact, to be touched and to touch their parents, if they are to develop and blossom fully. And if we are so reticent and reluctant about the idea of this contact even before trying it out, it is because we have been terribly deprived of these tactile exchanges by our educators, who were themselves prisoners of their Judeo-Christian guilt-ridden morality, putting shame on anything physical. How many times have some of us wished to be hugged by our fathers rather than just pecked with the tips of their lips on our forehead, or wished to be stroked, kneaded, massaged and pressed against their chests, instead of being held at a distance as if we had the plague?

This lack of physical contact is what is responsible for our inhibitions in this area, but it is not too late to re-learn to live out this sense banned by our parents. We can catch up for lost time and re-discover all our tactile possibilities and, above all, develop the neural connections within our central computer which are connected to the tips of our fingers.

And we must remember all this especially with our children, if we have any, and teach them to touch each other, to touch us and to be touched themselves.

MEDITATION 6 - EROTICISM AND MUTUAL EXCITEMENT

This CD or tape is designed to be listened to by two people who are considering having a sexual experience.

Our sexuality can be seen as the top of the tree's trunk which we are growing within us, from which stems the branches carrying the flowers of our total fulfilment and blossoming. A person cannot reach full awakening if their sexuality is not totally liberated and harmonious.

The physical union of two people is in fact the simplest action which requires the simultaneous use of the five senses, and moreover, is the easiest way to get in harmony with Infinity in a moment of total illumination, allowing us a glimpse of the state that we can be in permanently if we reach absolute awakening.

After the usual period of oxygenation which should always precede the playing of each CD and which aims to improve the quality of the chemical reactions within our brain, thus allowing us to feel what our five senses are picking up, the first part of this exercise consists of becoming visually aware of our partner's body.

Your partner is lying down next to you and you are looking at their physique from head to toe, becoming aware of this universe similar to yourself, with which you will soon be one and a part of, as two 'infinitely small', which are both part of the 'infinitely small', which are both part of the 'infinitely large', meet each other.

The one who is lying down, eyes closed, becomes aware of the other person's gaze caressing their body and 'feels it' moving along. Thus they are offering their charming body curves to the visual organs of the person with whom they shall be progressing together in the awakening of their sensuality. The person lying down almost feels penetrated by the looks which are flowing into them through all the pores of their skin.

The second part of this exercise consists of exciting the erogenous zones of your partner by massaging them far more lightly than in CD number five, with caresses designed to excite sexually the person being massaged.

Certain parts of the body should be stroked very lightly while others should be massaged much harder, bearing individual sensitivity in mind. It is very important that the one being massaged collaborates fully during this exercise by expressing what they like or like less and which parts they wish to be stroked gently and which parts to be stroked harder. In fact, though the main erogenous zones are the same for everyone, there are certain variations depending on the individual personality, so that some parts which do nothing for some people are particularly exciting for others. With practice, we will be able to discover all these variations which produce even better results and refine our stimulation of the other person's sensitive parts.

What is more, it is most important that the one being stroked informs the stroker very precisely about everything that they feel. Even the most minute of pleasurable sensations must be manifested clearly by little moans. This will have three effects: first, it will guide the massager's hands with more precision, then it will trigger a feeling of excitement in the masseur as they perceive the results of the movements, and finally it will improve the quality of pleasure in the one being massaged through a process of positive feedback. The act of hearing yourself moaning with pleasure will trigger in your brain certain mechanisms which provoke an improvement in the functioning of the receptor organs. Pleasure generates pleasure, which is why it is most important to react to the slightest pleasurable sensation at the beginning of the exercise by moaning loud enough for your partner to perceive the pleasurable sensations, by slightly amplifying the vocal manifestations of these positive perceptions, even if, to begin with, the sensations were not quite large enough to push you to express your satisfaction audibly. This amplification of our reactions to pleasure will produce an amplification of the pleasure itself.

Once our sense of vision, touch and hearing has been in contact with our partner, now the sense of taste and smell can come into action.

This time the same areas which have just been stroked with the tips of the fingers will now be touched gently with the lips, tasted with the tip of the tongue in some areas, and smelled and breathed upon in others, so that the person lying down feels the hot breath of the person who is discovering them through the nose and mouth. It is important during this exercise to breathe in through the nose so as to exercise the sense of smell and to breathe out through the mouth so that your partner lying down feels your breath on their skin. The discovery of body smells on your partner is very important. It has been scientifically proven that body smells contain certain chemicals called pheromones, a word coming from the Greek 'phe-rein' meaning 'carrier' and 'hormao' meaning 'I exist', thus together meaning 'I broadcast my existence'. The name was given to all sub-stances which are secreted by living organisms which influence the behaviour of others of the same species.

Certain moths can find their partners of the opposite sex during the mating season by tracing a smell emitted by the latter up to several kilometres away, even in a wood full of other smells. Thus we can understand just how important this sense is. What is more, certain cases of impotence have been cured by using the odours emitted by the female sexual organ and cases of frigidity by men's odours – yet another reason for not using deodorants if we wish to have an harmonious sexual life.

In addition, it is important to understand clearly that fresh body odours do not smell bad. Fresh sweat, for example, is not at all unpleasant to smell. If, on the other hand, we do not wash for a long time, and we allow the sweat to ferment on us and in our clothes, it becomes completely unbearable. Even roses begin to smell bad when they rot.

Thus we have just seen that certain substances contained in our body odours affect our sexual reactions. This is why it is vital to breathe in and smell our partner in the areas described by the CD and to allow these particular substances to produce their own exciting effects in our brain.

The same goes for the sense of taste. The skin secretes substances which also have their importance and which contain chemical messages which the receptors of our tongue decode and transmit to our brain, which itself relays other chemical and neural messages to our sexual organs so that they can prepare for action.

The exchange of breath is also essential since it allows both bodies to harmonize their breathing and to feel themselves living, thanks to the same rhythm.

Also, this air which has been in contact with the inside of our body takes up atoms which have travelled within us and contributes to the reciprocal 'connection' of the two organisms.

Finally, the kissing enables both people to exchange chemical messages by communicating with their taste buds, and to directly taste the other person tasting them with a similar organ. We cannot do this with hearing or smelling, but we can with touch when people are mutually touching each other with the tips of their fingers, but it is even more intense with the mouth.

At the end of this exercise it will be the turn of the other person who was lying down, to do on the other what the latter did for them. Thus both partners will at last be totally open to each other and ready to unite while bearing in mind the wondrous scale of this meeting of two universes, who are mutually enriching each other.

Reaching a conscious orgasm simultaneously, felt by the whole body rather than just by the sexual organs, will be the reward of scrupulous preparation of this celebration of Infinity, which could last a very long time and which will have nothing to do with what until now has been called 'making love'.

The absolute symbiosis of two people finally becoming a bit of each other allows them to make love with the atoms which make them up and with the galaxies of which they are part, and thus to have what can be called a cosmic orgasm.

7

THE CENTRES OF SENSUAL MEDITATION

The programme which we have just analyzed does not represent the totality of the teaching given to 'Man' by the 'watchmakers' who made us, but as stated above, it is the tree trunk of our fulfilment. A tree with just a trunk cannot live, and every branch is vital for the development of the leaves which allow it to breathe and for the flowers to blossom. The branches are other exercises which are just as important, but which were not able to be presented in the form of recorded CDs, because some necessitate the intervention of a teacher of Sensual Meditation (whom we call a guide), and others require the presence of a group as is the case, among others, for the development of the collective harmonic vocal vibration.

We could also mention as part of the process of awakening, the guided and progressive discovery of the beauty of our own body through an initiation into naturalism, allowing us to appreciate the beauty and harmony of every part of our body by comparing them with those of our course companions. This is particularly important for women in whom the idea has been inculcated that their sexual organ is dirty and ugly. By comparing this part of themselves with each other, they can discover how wonderfully interesting and full of grace their sexual organs are, in their innumerable variety of shapes.

Men, too, can forget their inferiority complexes by discovering the richness of their sexual organs, each marvellously adapted for relations with their partners. They can discover the great variety of shapes and sizes, each one with its own advantages and thus none of them inferior to any other.

But one of the most important groups of exercises consists of the improvement in the use of the senses, which are also developed in these centres. It is the development of the five basic senses which finally allows the development of the sixth one, that is to say, the ability to communicate telepathically. This last sense develops only when all the others are capable of functioning to their maximum potential.

This is a brief glimpse of the possibilities offered by these centres of Sensual Meditation which are truly schools of sensuality.

Moreover, it is important to note the utility of these centres for our youth – those adolescents whose parents do not dare explain the facts of life and whose educators present them with a 'sexual education' which talks only about dogs and mice. Basically, they explain only 'how it works' rather than teaching them how to use their organs to attain the maximum pleasure. They try to make out that sex is only for procreation, even though in our day and age our contraceptive techniques are improving all the time. We provide young girls with the 'pill', yet we tell them that sexual union is only for making babies, one of the heights of human hypocrisy.

These Sensual Meditation centres will be open only to those 'above the age of consent', which represents different ages depending on the legislation of the country in which the centre is located. In France, for example, you must be at least 18 years old to frequent the centres, and those between the ages of 15 and 18 require a written authorization from their parents, a draft form of which will be provided by our 'sensuality schools'. Those between the ages of 15 and 18 have the right (!) to have a sexual life with the consent (!) of their parents. As for those under the age of 15, even if their parents consent, they have no right to a sexual life. It is not our fault, it is the law!

Inform yourselves at your local Sensual Meditation centre which will let you know the current laws concerning the age limits of your country which we have to respect. If you are too young, be patient, and in the meantime awaken yourselves by yourselves, according to principles described in this book.

THE FUNCTION OF THE GUIDE

Though some particularly gifted individuals can learn how to awaken and blossom by themselves, most people would do better to be guided along the path of harmony so as to avoid wasting time along directions which lead to nothing. And even the particularly gifted people will still waste a lot of time with unproductive experiences unless they meet someone who will give them the benefit of their own experience.

Awakening has sometimes been compared to a mountain with many paths leading to the top, the attainment of which represents self-realization. Personally, I prefer comparing it to a tree which we cultivate within ourselves, and which is therefore different for each person, both in shape and in the fruit which it will produce. A mountain representing awakening would imply that there is only one summit to reach and everyone must climb the same mountain, which is incorrect, and even if we admitted that everyone has his or her own personal mountain, then that would mean that once we reach the top, there will be nothing left to discover. With the other image, the tree is alive and we never cease to develop it, growing its branches and bearing more and more fruit, the flavours of each one becoming more and more delicious.

That is why those who teach Sensual Meditation are, above all, gardeners, even though the only title which they would accept would be 'guides'. They are there to guide the saplings as they begin to grow, so that their development is as rapid and harmonious as can be.

A real guide will never accept being called 'master' since, deriving from the Latin word 'magister', its meaning is to have authority over people, and the guide is not there to order anyone around, but on the contrary, to allow the young tree to decide what is the right direction to send out its roots by letting it discover all its possibilities. And the best way to help it take the best possible decision is to allow it to develop its links connecting it with Infinity, that is to say, by developing its senses. We have seen that the word 'meditate' comes from the Latin word 'meditare' which means 'to exercise'. Therefore, Sensual Meditation is a training of the senses aimed at an improved perception of the Infinite, eventually allowing us to realize that we ourselves are infinite and leading us to develop completely naturally in the best possible direction.

When putting ourselves in harmony with the Infinite, we ourselves become the vehicle or instrument through which it is manifest in the eyes of those who are not yet aware of the Infinite.

The guide is no more than a manifestation of the Infinite, addressed to those who have not yet realized that they, too, can be the instrument of what they are made up of and what they make up.

Guides do not teach love, they are love because they derive their pleasure from seeing others develop, and are nourished by their progress.

They do not see people when they teach, they see only manifestations of Infinity whom they are helping to become aware of what and who they are.

The guides do not teach so as to be loved or admired, they teach so as to give to other bits of Infinity the joy of realizing what they are, because they admire in others that which animates themselves.

You who are reading these lines, you, too, are composed of Infinity which is in the process of discovering itself, and that is why you feel as enthusiastic as you do now. The guides are there to help you prolong and develop this enthusiasm.

The word 'enthusiasm' comes from the Greek word 'entheos' which means 'inspired by the Gods', and as we have seen, this concept of God represents infinity. Thus, to help you to be 'inspired by Infinity' which is you, that is the aim of the guide.

8

PERSONAL EXPERIENCES

Here are a few of the more notable personal experiences sent by some of the hundreds of people who have already followed a course of awakening through Sensual Meditation.

When I arrived at the site of the course of awakening on the 5th August I was still wondering what I was doing there, especially as I've always found it very hard to approach people.

Always ill at ease with myself, I had been carrying about for a couple of years then some badly healed emotional injuries which had made me retreat into my shell just like a snail which had been frightened. Relatively ignorant about the damage which can be caused by nastiness and stupidity, I discovered a few years beforehand the destructive power of words, and after having met shame, anxiety, fear and panic of other people, I was emotionally injured and had found refuge in my solitude.

It was in this state of mind that I came into contact with Rael and the Raelians; something very strong had pushed me there, but like a fighter on his guard, I was closed into myself, suspicious and tense.

The next day the course of awakening started and in the company of a few dozen men and women, we embarked upon a subject which for me required serious thinking and to which I had so far remained very painfully closed and sensitive: sexuality.

It was as if I was extracting from my flesh a foreign body which had been poisoning me, and as everyone expelled from themselves their own memories which had been poisoning them, so too did I start hearing myself relate in my shaky voice in a way that I would never have thought possible. I was feeling the support from the trust which had been built up so rapidly between us all, men and women, even though we had met each other only the previous evening. I had just discovered Raelian fraternity and rapport, something which, until then, I was unfamiliar with, and in front of them I had just got rid of a huge load which before, I had been trailing about with me for far too long.

And throughout the course, Rael had handled with simplicity, common sense and in-depth knowledge this subject for which in the past I had only heard derogatory laughter and rude remarks from others.

How can I describe all the benefits of this course without missing any out, apart from saying that it changed my life completely, not to mention all the deep changes of which I am not yet aware.

More open in mind and body, more aware of myself and others, little by little I have noticed that many things have changed in my outlook on life and in the way I live it.

The range of values which I had previously built up seemed outmoded and from that moment, I think, I started to consider other people and events with much more acuity and serenity, as if they had shed their deceitful facade and as if they had taken back their real dimensions.

I also rediscovered, I think, the capacity of my youth to marvel at everything and everyone as if seeing with new eyes, looking as if in love at women and at life in all its variety with an ever greater sensitivity.

This internal revolution also had its effects upon my way of behaving, a change which itself was not without its problems since, and this I realized straight away, my acquaintances could not or did not always try to understand why they found me as someone different to the person whom they knew before. I had to balance my desire to realize myself to the full, with the fear of shocking the people whom I love or whom I feel something for, and yet I still try to temper my way of being with common sense.

The final result is that those with whom I live see me in a new light; they are left both surprised and wondering and, in general, respect my way of being since it appeals to their reason, and from their attitude towards me, I believe that I am taken into more consideration, and people respect me more.

Rene Jourdren, Saint Etienne, France

Before participating in the course of awakening, my life didn't have the same intensity. In fact, I wasn't autonomous or independent and tended to solve my problems by leaning on others a lot. I would seek things which I didn't have without giving anything in exchange. I was caught in a system of consumerism. In the same way as a consumer needs to have things, I would swallow food and words, losing out on the meaning of dialogue, exchange and sharing.

Thanks to the course of awakening, I have experienced the importance of interchanges and interactions, these exchanges which make life possible. But for that it is necessary to know ourselves and to like ourselves for what we are. It's much simpler! 'If you like yourself even a little bit, then you'll like others.'

During this course of awakening, Rael gave us the basis of the awakening of our body and hence of our mind, by emphasizing the importance of breathing. This breathing allows us to communicate with the outside world. But that isn't all, our body possesses other senses which serve us every day and which we are not conscious of, yet if they didn't exist there wouldn't be any interaction between us and the outside world, and therefore no life.

Rael taught us how to utilize our senses sensually. This course of awakening is a birth into the senses which I attempt to live out every day. I can measure my development by the reactions of the people who surround me. People say to me: 'you create a feeling of confidence because you're always smiling.'

The course of awakening made me realize that life is not just a routine, but on the contrary, can be infinitely rich when we become one with it. Now I experience things in life as much outside me as inside me. Everything is simple. My life now contains only those interchanges and interactions which unite me in a beautiful harmony called love.

Chantal Lemetayer, Rennes, France

I used to stumble in the darkness, imprisoned by an atrophying education, colliding with all the taboos that centuries of obscurantism had imposed through the ages.

And yet one fine day the sun rose as I discovered Sensual Meditation during a 'course of awakening' supervised by Rael For me, it was the dawn of a new life. Up till then, all my shutters were closed, but at that moment, they opened onto a beautiful landscape. I had rediscovered the secrets of my body.

It is very difficult to describe in words all the treasures that this brought me. Instead, I would rather that one day, everyone could live what I feel and experience through Sensual Meditation.

It was through this that I was able to rediscover simplicity, and that in everything, in every passing moment, there is an unlimited source of pleasure: the look of a child, the freshness of a summer's rain, a flower, a bird singing... In the same way that a bee creams the pollen from every flower, Sensual Meditation teaches us how to harvest the nectar of life with all the strength of our senses, from every moment of our existence.

And now every morning, while millions of people wake up into the monotony of habit, my mind awakes into a whirlwind of colours. An infinite energy rises from the depths of my brain and illuminates all of my cells. Imagination and creativity know no bounds, and sensuality takes the lead.

My body was the bud of a marvellous flower, which the shadows of civilization and religion prevented from growing. Sensual Meditation was the ray of sunshine, which made the bud blossom and opened it into the harmony of infinite space and time.

Pierre Gary, engineer, Paris

I am 16 years old and my name is Laurence. I discovered Sensual Meditation and it was a revelation for me, something very powerful, burning me like a voluptuous caress. Even more, it was ecstasy. Yet I had been doing yoga for many years, but it was nowhere near the same. I felt in perfect harmony with the whole of my body, the whole of my being and with other people. Your voice, recorded on the cassette, penetrated me right to my depth, every little part of my body was invaded by warmth. I was drunk with happiness and love. I would get up effortlessly after meditating as if floating, bathing or being carried by air, and it's the most beautiful thing that there is, to feel thus in harmony with everything that surrounds us.

On Sunday, I went to the Cevennes and I climbed very high up a mountain with a tape recorder and your cassette.

And there I lay down, facing the sky and its immensity... What words can I use to describe how I felt? No word is powerful enough or sensual enough to describe this feeling of being high. I used to smoke hashish before and take amphetamines to give me the illusion of being, of feeling good, but if you only knew how these drugs seem ridiculous now! I also stopped all that because it is completely unnecessary now that I have discovered Sensual Meditation. I have discovered an ideal, I breathe, I live, I exist, and I realize that only now.

I am learning to look at things in a better way, at flowers, and sometimes, it happens that I talk with a flower and am ecstatic over its beauty. There, time no longer exists, it is Infinity.

Laurence, Avignon, France

After the time spent practising the meditation this summer at the course of awakening, I now feel a new clarity of mind with an improved awareness of my personality, and therefore of my potential.

What is more, I have also noticed an improvement in my general well-being. I am lightly handicapped by a stiff spine, especially in the lumbar region. Since practising Sensual Meditation, I can feel a definite increase in suppleness in this area. It might be due purely to the breathing exercises which precede each meditation, but whatever the cause, I felt I had to give my testimony.

Pierre-Simon, Rennes, France

It is with immense joy that I wish to thank you Rael, for the unforgettable moments which we lived with you at the course of the 'awakening of the mind and body'. What transformed me the most was the moment where we created the void for a better 'renaissance' afterwards. I experienced such a strong emotion, that I wanted to shout my joy to everyone, but the emotion left me speechless. Since then, I feel as if a new man, I am starting my life afresh at 67 years old.

Alexandre-Denis, Saint Ubald, Canada

Since I am already of a certain age, my development following the course of awakening has occurred slowly, but surely. The change, however, certainly was radical since my associate asked me what was happening. Now that I have this feeling of joy within me, I must say that I have a thirst to live as long as possible and I have noticed that the more time passes, the more the meditation transforms me. For me, there is no greater joy than to be Raelian and my convictions are unshakable. I am sincere, and I have found what I was looking for after so many years.

Simone David, Montreal, Canada

When I first came across Rael and the teachings of our creators, the Elohim, my life was just a huge question mark. I was almost ashamed to be a man and I did not have the courage to face the prospect, on the one hand, of the social – economic – political – mystical – fanatical orgy, on which I was unable to open any doors without taking a beating, and on the other hand, that of the primitive obscurantism in which I had been immersed since my birth, and whose cast was stuck to my skin and would have asphyxiated me.

Despite everything, I was looking for something else, something which would allow me to breathe in peace, something logical, real and humane.

At the time I was timid, ill at ease and could not express myself, even in front of only one person. What is more, my sensual tastes required me to fulfil my senses with the contact of male bodies. Therefore, I was traumatized, and filled with guilt, I was disgraced by conventional morality, by religion, by education and by the most futile of simple customs.

Maybe you don't realize it, but one is born as a homosexual, just as one is born with green eyes or will inevitably have size 38 in shoes, or measure 1,42 metres, etc... that is to say, that in one's chromosomes, within the nucleus of an individual's cells, the stack of genes carries the characteristics of each person and determines absolutely everything about their tastes, shapes and everything which makes them original.

What is scandalous, is that in the middle ages they killed hysterics and not so long ago, they put heretics to death with the blessing of the obscurantist religions, and now of course, it is fashionable to kill political dissidents and homosexuals, whom they lock up in concentration camps, pompously called asylums or adjustment houses. Even in Paris, homosexuals are imprisoned, tortured, harassed, hemmed in, and forced to live underground in ghettos by this ignorant society and submit to this injustice. And yet, it is so easy to understand how such characteristics are determined genetically, thanks to the work of our scientists.

So, in the two years since I have known and practised Rael's teachings, I have seen myself totally transformed. I have now, little by little, discovered all my possibilities which I do not yet exploit completely, but at least I have discovered them and I am setting off on the exploitation of myself through the awakening of my faculties, just as a gardener who discovers his land, starts working the land to bring out its best before sowing, cultivating and finally harvesting.

All cultivation requires various technical knowledge, a bit of experience and a lot of common sense. Rael's teachings are a bit like that! To begin with, one must have the wish to open one's garden and to see it blossom with the most magnificent of plants, flowers and trees. The technical know-how is needed to clear the soil which has never been exploited, to liberate it from the weeds, the brambles and excess limestone, so as to regain a neutral environment, not too acid, not too alkaline and to restore a little order, just what is necessary so that what is desired can grow in the harmony of its climate and the richness of the soil.

The common sense is needed so as not to put the cart before the horse, so as to gauge what the soil can produce and at what rhythm, what it needs and what it has too much of, so that the balance can be restored at any time, under the watchful eye of the gardener.

The practical experience allows us to see how the soil is biological, full of natural chemicals. Just as we breathe, it is quite obvious that the Earth is alive, from the carrot and dandelion to 'Man', everything has its own specific function to fulfil, determined by each individual's genetic code contained within his or her cells. Every living thing is a cog in the harmonious equilibrium of the whole planet, each thing is finely tuned to everything else and only 'Man' is capable of understanding all this. Today, I live out my sexuality by seeking fulfilment through all my senses, and with whom I please. I now feel good with myself, my timidity is disappearing and as a consequence, my aggression is controlled.

Moreover, I am giving lectures to audiences of more than 100 people, I can now address myself to anyone, with total simplicity and more open-mindedness and respect for others. I can feel an infinity of dormant potential being awakened within me, the rhythm of exploitation which I can control, since it is precisely this control and management of each action, based on a mature awareness of each thought, felt by optimum functioning of the brain drawn away from its lethargy by the exercising of one's sensuality, that is one of the main qualities of Sensual Meditation.

I forgot to mention that since 1967, I have had a gastric ulcer, which at the time, I was advised to have operated on through surgery, but I refused in favour of a homeopathic treatment which I tried for the next 10 years, but without success. When I started practising Sensual Meditation, I still had the ulcer, but within a few months, it disappeared so completely that I even forgot to mention it. I have all the x- ray photos and medical certificates available for all sceptics to see, as well as my military service papers which, to my joy, certify me inept for service precisely because of my ulcer.

Michel Vuaillat, horticultural technician

I am 24 years old, and though I started my sexual life at 16 I've been frigid for the last eight years. That is, I made love, with the only pleasure being the contemplation of the effect of my body, which is of nice proportions, on my male partners.

I was limited to the pleasure of giving them pleasure, and like many women, I pretended to enjoy it so that they would feel virile, and so that I would not seem abnormal.

When I discovered Sensual Meditation at 24 years of age, I had my first orgasm. I put into words how beautiful this revelation was for me. I might add that I used to suffer regularly from bouts of depression and anxiety which no medication was able to cure, but which have now disappeared totally following this discovery of physical pleasure. I express one wish, and that is for every woman to be able to discover this, especially as I have learned that 70 per cent of women have never experienced an orgasm.

N.C., Quebec

I feel as if I have now discovered the source of pleasure, of happiness, and can draw pleasure from it at will.

Cristiane Gariepy, Montreal, Canada

BIBLIOGRAPHY

- Art et science de la creative, Publication du Centre culturel de Cerisy-la-Salle Published in the collection 10/18 by Union Generale d'Editions

- Evolution ou Creation by Jean Fiori Published by Editions S.D.T., 77190 Dammarlie-les-Lys, France

- L'orgasme au Feminin Published by Editions Univers, 1651 Saint-Denis, Montreal, Canada.

- Submission to Authority S. Milgram, Paris 1974

ADDITIONAL INFORMATION

The Sensual Meditation CDs and audio tapes and the poster of the symbol of Infinity can be obtained from the Raelian Movement of your country as on page 135 or ordered directly form the internet at www.rael.org

The official internet addresses of the Raelian Movement and associated organisations are: www.rael.org

To subscribe to rael-science, which distributes by e-mail a selection of scientific news concerning this book, in English, please send a blank e-mail to subscribe@rael-science.org

OTHE BOOKS BY RAEL

INTELLIGENT DESIGN: Message from the Designers
Years ago, everybody *knew* that the earth was flat. Everybody *knew* that the sun revolved around the earth. Today, everybody *knows* that life on earth is either the result of random evolution or the work of a supernatural God. Or is it?

In "Message from the Designers", Rael presents us with a third option: that all life on earth was created by advanced scientists from another world. During a UFO encounter in 1973, he was given the first of a series of messages, face to face, by one of these designers. Those messages now lie within the pages of this book - an astonishing revelation for mankind.

GENIOCRACY
The first English translation of a highly controversial political thesis
Democracy is an imperfect form of government destined to give way to rule by geniuses - "Geniocracy". Under this system, no candidate for high office may stand for election unless his intelligence level is measurably fifty per cent above the norm. Furthermore, to be eligible to vote, an elector must have an intelligence level ten per cent above the average. Geniocracy is, therefore, selective democracy.

These challenging concepts already apply on the planet of the Elohim. Unless we can come up with something better, they advise us to begin preparing to implement a similar system, since all human progress is ultimately dependent on the work of geniuses.

In this first edition of the book to be published in the English language, Rael describes how such a process might work here - once intelligence testing is sufficiently developed.

YES TO HUMAN CLONING
An amazing glimpse into the future
In this book, Rael, who inspired Clonaid, the first company offering to clone human beings, explains how today's technology is the first step in the quest for eternal life.

With exceptional vision, he allows us an extraordinary glimpse into an amazing future and explains how our nascent technology will revolutionize our world and transform our lives.

This is a book to prepare us for an unimaginably beautiful world turned paradise, where nanotechnology will make agriculture and heavy industry redundant, where super artificial intelligence will quickly outstrip human intelligence and do all the boring tasks, where eternal life will be just as possible in a computer as in a series of constantly rejuvenated human bodies, and where the world could be a place of leisure and love where no one need work no more!

THE MAITREYA
Extracts from his Teachings
Rael, the predicted "Maitreya from the West", shares his teachings and insights in this wonderful book of extracts taken from the many Raelian seminars at which he has taught over the past thirty years. A multitude of topics are covered in this book, such as Love, Happiness, Serenity, Spirituality, Contemplation, The Myth of Perfection, Non-Violence, Science, Loving Relationships, and much more. An excellent resource for anyone interested in developing oneself and wishing to live a more fulfilling and joyful life.

CD RECORDINGS

98

SENSUAL MEDITATION

The full set of six guided meditations from the book Sensual Meditation is available on two CDs or one audio tape cassette. The first and most important meditation 'Harmonization with Infinity' is available on a separate CD or tape. These can be ordered from the Raelian Movement of your country.

NARRATION OF THE BOOK

The Message Given By Extra-Terrestrials also exists as a fully narrated recording in 6 CDs

SEMINARS AND CONTACTS

Each year several seminars are held around the world where Raelians gather to hear the teachings of the Elohim as given by their Prophet Rael. If you would like to participate in one of these seminars or just get in touch with a Raelian near you, please contact one of the local Raelian Movements below. For a complete list of Raelian contacts in over 86 countries, please visit the website: **www.rael.org**

AFRICA
05 BP 1444, Abidjan 05
Ivory Coast
Africa
Tel: (+225) 07.82.83.00
E-mail: africa@intelligentdesignbook.com

AMERICA
P.O. Box 570935
Topaz Station
Las Vegas, NV
89108
USA
Tel: (+1) 888 RAELIAN / (+1) 888 723 5426
E-mail: usa@intelligentdesignbook.com
E-mail: canada@intelligentdesignbook.com

ASIA
Desukatto Shinjuku Nishiguchi Ten MB6
Matsuoka Central Bldg. 3F
Tokyo-To, Shinjuku-Ku
Nishi-Shinjuku 1-7-1
Japan 160-0023
Tel: (+81)3 5348 3866
Fax: (+81)3 5348 3910
E-mail: asia@intelligentdesignbook.com

EUROPE
P.O. Box 176
1926 Fully
Switzerland
Tel: +41 27 746 30 20
E-mail: europe@intelligentdesignbook.com

MIDDLE-EAST
P.O.Box 25415
Tel Aviv 61253
IsRael
Tel : +972 3 699 9869
E-mail: middle-east@intelligentdesignbook.com

OCEANIA
P.O. Box 2387, Fountain Gate
Vic, 3805
Australia
Tel: +61(0)409 376 544
Tel: +61(0)419 966 196
E-mail: oceania@intelligentdesignbook.com